T0226830

Melanoma

Editor

ADAM C. BERGER

SURGICAL ONCOLOGY
CLINICS OF NORTH AMERICA

www.surgonc.theclinics.com

Consulting Editor
NICHOLAS J. PETRELLI

April 2015 • Volume 24 • Number 2

ELSEVIER

1600 John F. Kennedy Boulevard • Suite 1800 • Philadelphia, Pennsylvania, 19103-2899

http://www.theclinics.com

SURGICAL ONCOLOGY CLINICS OF NORTH AMERICA Volume 24, Number 2
April 2015 ISSN 1055-3207, ISBN-13: 978-0-323-35987-0

Editor: Jessica McCool
Developmental Editor: Meredith Clinton

Surgical Oncology Clinics of North America (ISSN 1055-3207) is published quarterly by Elsevier Inc., 360 Park Avenue South, New York, NY 10010-1710. Months of publication are January, April, July, and October. Business and Editorial Offices: 1600 John F. Kennedy Blvd., Ste. 1800, Philadelphia, PA 19103-2899. Customer Service Office: 3251 Riverport Lane, Maryland Heights, MO 63043. Periodicals postage paid at New York, NY and additional mailing offices. Subscription prices are $290.00 per year (US individuals), $421.00 (US institutions) $140.00 (US student/resident), $330.00 (Canadian individuals), $533.00 (Canadian institutions), $205.00 (Canadian student/resident), $410.00 (foreign individuals), $533.00 (foreign institutions), and $205.00 (foreign student/resident). Foreign air speed delivery is included in all *Clinics* subscription prices. All prices are subject to change without notice. **POSTMASTER:** Send address changes to *Surgical Oncology Clinics of North America*, Elsevier Health Science Division, Subscription Customer Service, 3251 Riverport Lane, Maryland Heights, MO 63043. **Customer Service: 1-800-654-2452 (US and Canada). 314-447-8871 (outside US and Canada). Fax: 314-447-8029.** E-mail: journalscustomerservice-usa@elsevier.com (for print support); **journalsonline support-usa@elsevier.com** (for online support).

Reprints. For copies of 100 or more, of articles in this publication, please contact the Commercial Reprints Department, Elsevier Inc., 360 Park Avenue South, New York, New York 10010-1710. Tel. 212-633-3874; Fax: 212-633-3820; E-mail: reprints@elsevier.com.

Surgical Oncology Clinics of North America is covered in *MEDLINE/PubMed (Index Medicus)* and *EMBASE/ Excerpta Medica, Current Contents/Clinical Medicine, and ISI/BIOMED.*

Contributors

CONSULTING EDITOR

NICHOLAS J. PETRELLI, MD, FACS
Bank of America Endowed Medical Director, Helen F. Graham Cancer Center and Research Institute, Christiana Care Health System, Newark, Delaware; Professor of Surgery, Thomas Jefferson University, Philadelphia, Pennsylvania

EDITOR

ADAM C. BERGER, MD, FACS
Professor, Chief, Section of Surgical Oncology, Department of Surgery, Thomas Jefferson University, Philadelphia, Pennsylvania

AUTHORS

CHARLOTTE ARIYAN, MD, PhD
Assistant Attending, Memorial Sloan Kettering Cancer Center, New York, New York

EDMUND K. BARTLETT, MD
Department of Surgery, University of Pennsylvania, Philadelphia, Pennsylvania

JANICE N. CORMIER, MD, MPH
Professor, Department of Surgical Oncology, The University of Texas MD Anderson Cancer Center, Houston, Texas

KATE D. CROMWELL, MS, MPH
Clinical Studies Coordinator, Department of Surgical Oncology, The University of Texas MD Anderson Cancer Center, Houston, Texas

KEITH A. DELMAN, MD
Associate Professor, Division of Surgical Oncology, Department of Surgery, Winship Cancer Institute-Emory University, Atlanta, Georgia

GARY B. DEUTSCH, MD
John Wayne Cancer Institute, Providence St. John's Hospital, Santa Monica, California

MAGGIE L. DILLER, MD
Division of Surgical Oncology, Department of Surgery, Winship Cancer Institute-Emory University, Atlanta, Georgia

MATTHEW P. DOEPKER, MD
Department of Cutaneous Oncology, Moffitt Cancer Center, Tampa, Florida

DAVID E. ELDER, MB ChB, FRCPA
Professor, Department of Pathology and Laboratory Medicine, Hospital of the University of Pennsylvania, Philadelphia, Pennsylvania

MARK B. FARIES, MD, FACS
John Wayne Cancer Institute, Providence St. John's Hospital, Santa Monica, California

JEFFREY M. FARMA, MD
Department of Surgical Oncology, Fox Chase Cancer Center, Philadelphia, Pennsylvania

KENDRA J. FEENEY, MD
Clinical Assistant Professor, Department of Medical Oncology, Sidney Kimmel School of Medicine, Thomas Jefferson University, Philadelphia, Pennsylvania

JAMIE GREEN, MD
Research Fellow, Memorial Sloan Kettering Cancer Center, New York, New York

CARY HSU, MD
Divisions of General Surgery and Surgical Oncology, Department of Surgery, David Geffen School of Medicine at UCLA, Los Angeles, California

GIORGOS C. KARAKOUSIS, MD
Assistant Professor, Department of Surgery, University of Pennsylvania, Philadelphia, Pennsylvania

DANIEL D. KIRCHOFF, MD
John Wayne Cancer Institute, Providence St. John's Hospital, Santa Monica, California

NANDINI KULKARNI, MD
Department of Surgical Oncology, Fox Chase Cancer Center, Philadelphia, Pennsylvania

BENJAMIN M. MARTIN, MD
Division of Surgical Oncology, Department of Surgery, Winship Cancer Institute-Emory University, Atlanta, Georgia

MICHAEL J. MASTRANGELO, MD
Professor, Department of Medical Oncology, Sidney Kimmel School of Medicine, Thomas Jefferson University, Philadelphia, Pennsylvania

CLAIRE H. MERIWETHER, BA
Department of Surgery, Duke University Medical Center, Durham, North Carolina

STERGIOS J. MOSCHOS, MD
Clinical Associate Professor, Division of Hematology/Oncology, Department of Medicine, University of North Carolina at Chapel Hill, Chapel Hill, North Carolina

RAMYA PINNAMANENI, MD
Clinical Fellow, Division of Hematology/Oncology, Department of Medicine, East Carolina University, Greenville, North Carolina

NATASHA M. RUETH, MD, MS
Fellow, Department of Surgical Oncology, The University of Texas MD Anderson Cancer Center, Houston, Texas

WENYIN SHI, MD, PhD
Department of Radiation Oncology, Thomas Jefferson University, Philadelphia, Pennsylvania

PAUL J. SPEICHER, MD
Resident, Department of Surgery, Duke University Medical Center, Durham, North Carolina

DOUGLAS S. TYLER, MD
John Woods Harris Distinguished Professor and Chairman, Department of Surgery, University of Texas Medical Branch, Galveston, Texas

JONATHAN S. ZAGER, MD, FACS
Director of Regional Therapies; Chair of Graduate Medical Education, Department of Cutaneous Oncology, Moffitt Cancer Center, Tampa, Florida

Contents

Foreword: Melanoma   xiii

Nicholas J. Petrelli

Preface: Melanoma   xv

Adam C. Berger

Erratum   xvii

Current Staging and Prognostic Factors in Melanoma   215

Edmund K. Bartlett and Giorgos C. Karakousis

> The current American Joint Commission for Cancer staging system for melanoma includes thickness, ulceration, and mitotic index as primary tumor factors for patients with stage I and II disease. Number and size of nodal metastases, presence of satellitosis and in-transit disease, and tumor ulceration status categorize patients with stage III disease. Presence and location of distant metastatic disease and increased lactate dehydrogenase level stratify prognosis in patients with stage IV disease. Factors predictive of sentinel lymph node positivity are also studied, particularly in patients with T1 melanomas, but are not always congruent with those predictive of survival.

Pathology of Melanoma   229

David E. Elder

> The pathology of melanoma is discussed in relation to surgical diagnosis and management. Pitfalls that may result in problems of clinicopathologic communication are emphasized. A compelling vision for the future is that all tumors will be characterized by their driving oncogenes, suppressor genes, and other genomic factors. The success of targeted therapy directed against individual oncogenes, despite its limitations, suggests that a repertoire of targeted agents will be developed that can be used against a variety of different tumors, depending on the results of genetic testing. Nevertheless, histopathologic diagnosis and surgical therapy will remain mainstays of management for melanoma.

Surgical Management of Primary and Recurrent Melanoma   239

Jeffrey M. Farma, Nandini Kulkarni, and Cary Hsu

> Melanoma accounts for less than 2% of skin cancer cases but causes most skin cancer–related deaths. Surgery continues to be the cornerstone of treatment of melanoma and surgical principles are guided by data derived from clinical research. This article examines the evolution of surgical techniques for the diagnosis and treatment of primary and locally recurrent melanoma.

Sentinel Lymph Node Mapping in Melanoma in the Twenty-first Century   249

Matthew P. Doepker and Jonathan S. Zager

The incidence of melanoma is increasing faster than any other cancer. The status of the regional nodal basin remains the most important prognostic factor. Sentinel lymph node biopsy (SLNB) is recommended for staging in patients diagnosed with intermediate-thickness melanoma (1.01–4.0 mm). SLNB is considered somewhat controversial, especially when used to stage thin (1 mm), thick (>4 mm), or desmoplastic melanoma. This article reviews the current literature regarding SLNB in thin, intermediate, thick, and desmoplastic melanoma. Data supporting the use of newer radiopharmaceuticals in sentinel lymph node mapping along with newer imaging modalities are also reviewed.

Lymph Node Dissection for Stage III Melanoma   261

Maggie L. Diller, Benjamin M. Martin, and Keith A. Delman

Locoregional spread of melanoma to its draining lymph node basin is the strongest negative prognostic factor for patients. Exclusive of clinical trials, patients with sentinel lymph node–positive (microscopic) or clinically palpable (macroscopic) nodal disease should undergo lymphadenectomy. This article reviews the management and technical aspects of surgical care for regional metastases. Adjunct therapies (immunotherapy, targeted therapy, and radiation) may supplement lymphadenectomy in certain patient populations. Surgical morbidity after lymphadenectomy can be substantial, creating opportunities for improvement via minimally invasive techniques or refined patient selection.

Metastasectomy for Stage IV Melanoma   279

Gary B. Deutsch, Daniel D. Kirchoff, and Mark B. Faries

Metastatic melanoma has an unpredictable natural history but a predictably high mortality. Despite recent advances in systemic therapy, many patients do not respond, or develop resistance to drug therapy. Surgery has consistently shown good outcomes in appropriately selected patients. It is likely to be even more successful in the era of more effective medical treatment. Surgery should remain a strongly considered option for metastatic melanoma.

Intralesional Therapy for In-transit and Satellite Metastases in Melanoma   299

Kendra J. Feeney and Michael J. Mastrangelo

Intratumoral therapy with bacteria/bacterial products dates to at least the 1890s. Over the decades this has expanded beyond the use of microbes and microbial products to include chemicals, cancer chemotherapeutic agents, cytokines, recombinant organisms, and hybrid molecules. The appeal of this method of delivery is the ability to deliver high concentrations of the therapeutic agent directly to the tumor, often with minimal side effects. This article summarizes the use and efficacy of the various agents used in the past and present in the treatment of in-transit and satellite metastases in melanoma.

Regional Therapies for In-transit Disease 309

Paul J. Speicher, Claire H. Meriwether, and Douglas S. Tyler

In-transit melanoma is an uncommon pattern of recurrence, but presents unique management challenges and opportunities for treatment. The clinical presentation usually involves from 1 to more than 100 small subcutaneous or cutaneous nodules, ranging from submillimeter to multiple centimeters in diameter. Regional chemotherapy techniques are a mainstay of treatment of patients without systemic disease spread. Future applications of regional therapy are likely to involve combination therapy with cytotoxic agents and novel immune modulators. Regional therapy provides distinct opportunities for the treatment of unresectable disease, and offers a unique platform for investigation of novel therapeutics in early-stage clinical trials.

Role for Radiation Therapy in Melanoma 323

Wenyin Shi

Although melanoma is generally considered a relative radioresistant tumor, radiation therapy (RT) remains a valid and effective treatment option in definitive, adjuvant, and palliative settings. Definitive RT is generally only used in inoperable patients. Despite a high-quality clinical trial showing adjuvant RT following lymphadenectomy in node-positive melanoma patients prevents local and regional recurrence, the role of adjuvant RT in the treatment of melanoma remains controversial and is underused. RT is highly effective in providing symptom palliation for metastatic melanoma. RT combined with new systemic options, such as immunotherapy, holds promise and is being actively evaluated.

Update on Immunotherapy in Melanoma 337

Jamie Green and Charlotte Ariyan

Immunotherapy is now recognized as a viable option for patients with metastatic melanoma. The field of immunotherapy now offers treatments with the potential for a long-term cure. As the field moves forward, studies will focus on improving the response rates with new immunotherapy agents or novel treatment combinations.

Targeted Therapies in Melanoma 347

Stergios J. Moschos and Ramya Pinnamaneni

Advances in the biology of melanoma have provided insights about chemoresistance and its genetic heterogeneity in parallel with advances in drug design, culminating in recent major treatment breakthroughs. Although clinical benefit of targeted therapies has been unquestionable, future advances are only possible if we understand the interplay between genetic aberrations and role of other crucial nongenetic changes yet to be identified by such projects as the Cancer Genome Atlas Project in Melanoma. Combination therapies, either among small molecule inhibitors themselves and/or with immunotherapies, may be the optimal strategy to prevent development of drug resistance inherently linked with such targeted therapies.

Long-term Follow-up for Melanoma Patients: Is There Any Evidence of a Benefit?   359

Natasha M. Rueth, Kate D. Cromwell, and Janice N. Cormier

As the incidence of melanoma and the number of melanoma survivors continues to rise, optimal surveillance strategies are needed that balance the risks and benefits of screening in the context of contemporary resource use. Detection of recurrences has important implications for clinical management. Most current surveillance recommendations for melanoma survivors are based on low-level evidence with wide variations in practice patterns and an unknown clinical impact for the melanoma survivor.

SURGICAL ONCOLOGY
CLINICS OF NORTH AMERICA

FORTHCOMING ISSUES

July 2015
Head and Neck Cancer
John A. Ridge, *Editor*

October 2015
Genetic Testing and its Surgical Oncology Implications
Thomas Weber, *Editor*

January 2016
Endocrine Tumors
Douglas L. Fraker, *Editor*

RECENT ISSUES

January 2015
Hepatocellular Cancer, Cholangiocarcinoma, and Metastatic Tumors of the Liver
Lawrence P. Wagman, *Editor*

October 2014
Imaging in Oncology
Vijay Khatri, *Editor*

July 2014
Breast Cancer
Lisa A. Newman, *Editor*

RELATED INTEREST

Surgical Clinics of North America, October 2014 (Vol. 94, Issue 5)
Melanoma
Kimberly M. Brown and Celia Chao, *Editors*
Available at: http://www.surgical.theclinics.com/

DOWNLOAD
Free App!

Review Articles
THE CLINICS

NOW AVAILABLE FOR YOUR iPhone and iPad

Foreword

Melanoma

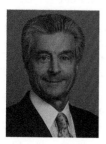

Nicholas J. Petrelli, MD, FACS
Consulting Editor

This issue of the *Surgical Oncology Clinics of North America* covers the topic of melanoma. The guest editor is Adam Berger, MD, FACS, who is the Chief of the Section of Surgical Oncology in the Department of Surgery at Thomas Jefferson University. In 2015, there will be approximately 76,000 new cases of melanoma with over 9,000 deaths. In our own state of Delaware, melanoma is one of the higher-incidence cancers because of the beautiful beaches in the southern part of the state. Educational efforts continue in our state concerning the dangers of sunlight and tanning beds. Teenagers don't realize that the use of tanning beds before the age of 35 increases the risk of melanoma by 75%. Recently, a law was passed in our state that requires parents' permission for a child under the age of 18 to utilize a tanning bed. It is not ideal, but it is a start. We continue to educate the public about the dangers of sunlight and tanning beds because melanoma is a preventable cancer.

Dr Berger has gathered an outstanding group of authors on the subject matter of the diagnosis and treatment of melanoma. This issue runs the gamut of melanoma from staging and prognostic factors to treatment, including targeted therapies and an update on immunotherapy. The last issue of the *Surgical Oncology Clinics of North America* dealing with melanoma was in January of 2011, and the guest editor was Jeffrey E. Gershenwald, MD, FACS, Professor in the Department of Surgical Oncology and Department of Cancer Biology at the University of Texas MD Anderson Cancer Center. In four short years, as demonstrated by this issue of the *Surgical Oncology Clinics of North America*, much progress has been made in the treatment of malignant melanoma. Hence, this issue is excellent timing.

Surg Oncol Clin N Am 24 (2015) xiii–xiv
http://dx.doi.org/10.1016/j.soc.2015.01.002
1055-3207/15/$ – see front matter © 2015 Elsevier Inc. All rights reserved.

surgonc.theclinics.com

I would like to thank Dr Berger for this timely issue of the *Surgical Oncology Clinics of North America*, and as I have said numerous times before, it is important that attending staff share this issue with all of their trainees.

Nicholas J. Petrelli, MD, FACS
Bank of America Endowed Medical Director
Helen F Graham Cancer Center & Research Institute
Christiana Care Health Systems
4701 Ogletown Stanton Road, Suite 1233
Newark, DE 19713, USA

Professor of Surgery
Thomas Jefferson University
Philadelphia, PA 19107, USA

E-mail address:
npetrelli@christianacare.org

Preface
Melanoma

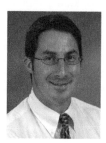

Adam C. Berger, MD, FACS
Editor

Although malignant melanoma accounts for only a small percentage (~2%) of all skin cancers, it is responsible for the vast majority of deaths. In 2015, it is estimated that around 76,000 new cases of melanoma will be diagnosed, and the number of new cases has been increasing every year for the last decade. Up to 80% of patients are diagnosed with early-stage disease (stages 0, 1, and 2) and are treated and cured surgically. However, there are still many patients presenting with stage 3 and 4 disease, which are much more difficult to surgically cure, and other therapies are essential. In addition, we are, increasingly, realizing that many patients with stage 1 and 2 disease will eventually develop metastatic disease, at which point treatment and cure are more difficult. Luckily, in the past few years, we have seen FDA approval of several new agents for the treatment of patients with metastatic melanoma, including targeted agents (Zelbroaf, Mekinist) and immune checkpoint blockade agents (Yervoy, Keytruda), which have dramatically changed the landscape for now and the future.

In this issue of *Surgical Oncology Clinics of North America*, we aim to highlight advances in the treatment of melanoma in the last five years. Any publication discussing the treatment of melanoma would be remiss in not acknowledging the seminal role of Dr Donald Morton, who sadly passed away during the production of this issue. Dr Morton played a seminal role in the development of the field of melanoma surgical oncology with his pioneering studies on sentinel lymph node mapping and biopsy as well as vaccine therapies and metastasectomy for patients with stage IV disease. In addition, he trained many of the current leaders in the field. We will surely miss his wonderful insights and contributions.

In the first article, Dr Edmund Bartlett and Dr Giorgos Karakousis have outlined the important changes to the 7th edition of the AJCC staging manual for melanoma, including relevant prognostic factors and the importance of mitotic rate. Dr David Elder, a well-known pathologist, provides an excellent primer on melanoma pathology

Surg Oncol Clin N Am 24 (2015) xv–xvi
http://dx.doi.org/10.1016/j.soc.2015.01.001
1055-3207/15/$ – see front matter © 2015 Published by Elsevier Inc.

surgonc.theclinics.com

in the second article. He presents important information regarding various subtypes of melanoma and describes important immunohistochemical and molecular diagnostic information. The surgical treatment of primary melanoma, including a breakdown on surgical margins, is provided by Dr Jeffrey Farma and his colleagues at Fox Chase Cancer Center. I have also asked him to discuss the treatment of locally recurrent melanoma. Dr Jonathan Zager gives an excellent breakdown on the importance of sentinel node biopsy for patients with melanoma, including in those with thin and thick lesions. He also describes some newer and more sophisticated imaging and mapping techniques. Radical lymph node dissections for patients with clinically positive or sentinel node–positive lymph nodes are outlined in detail by Keith Delman and his colleagues at Emory. They provide wonderful descriptions and figures in this article.

The next six articles primarily concern those patients who have developed metastatic disease. Dr Mark Faries, a disciple of Dr Morton, gives a systematic review of the rationale for surgical therapy for patients with metastatic disease. This is followed by two articles concerning the treatment of patients with unresectable satellite and in-transit recurrences, which are confined to the extremities. One of the leaders in the surgical field, Dr Douglas Tyler, gives an excellent overview of isolated limb perfusion and infusion, including his group's attempts to push the envelope with newer targeted agents. On the other hand, my colleagues, Dr Kendra Feeney and Dr Mike Mastrangelo, provide an excellent treatise on injectional and local therapy, including TVEC, which has had promising results in recent clinical trials. Dr Wenyin Shi supplies a nice summary of the use of radiation therapy for adjuvant therapy and treatment of metastatic disease, especially to the brain and spine. Finally, we have well-written reviews of systemic therapies by Dr Charlotte Ariyan from Sloan-Kettering (Immunotherapies) and Dr Stergios Moschos from UNC-Chapel Hill (Targeted therapies). In the final article, I have asked Dr Janice Cormier and her colleagues from MD Anderson to discuss evidence-based approaches to long-term follow-up of patients diagnosed with melanoma after their surgical therapy.

I would like to express my sincerest gratitude to all of those at Elsevier who have guided me through this process, including Jessica McCool, Meredith Clinton, and Stephanie Carter. I would also like to express my thanks to Dr Nicholas Petrelli for his invitation to serve as guest editor for this issue; I am truly honored to have this opportunity. My hope is that this issue of Surgical Oncology Clinics of North America provides an excellent reference and resource to those of us who are involved in the day-to-day care of patients with melanoma. It is hoped that it will spur the next generation of dedicated clinicians to new and exciting discoveries to further advances in this important field of study.

Adam C. Berger, MD, FACS
Section of Surgical Oncology
Department of Surgery
Thomas Jefferson University
Philadelphia, PA 19107, USA

E-mail address:
Adam.Berger@jefferson.edu

Erratum

In the October 2014 issue of *Surgical Oncology Clinics of North America*, Vol. 23, No. 4, Dr Fananapazir's name was spelled incorrectly on pages iv and 789 for the article "Diagnostic Imaging of Hepatic Lesions in Adults," by Ramit Lamba, Ghaneh Fananapazir, Michael T. Corwin, and Vijay P. Khatri. Fananapazir is the correct spelling.

Surg Oncol Clin N Am 24 (2015) xvii
http://dx.doi.org/10.1016/j.soc.2014.12.013
1055-3207/15/$ – see front matter © 2015 Elsevier Inc. All rights reserved.

surgonc.theclinics.com

Current Staging and Prognostic Factors in Melanoma

 CrossMark

Edmund K. Bartlett, MD, Giorgos C. Karakousis, MD*

KEYWORDS

• Melanoma • Staging • Prognosis • Sentinel lymph node • Prognostic factors

KEY POINTS

- In the current (seventh) edition of the American Joint Commission for Cancer staging system, tumor thickness, ulceration status, and mitotic index categorize patients with stage I and II melanoma.
- Size (micro vs macro), number of nodal metastases, presence of satellitosis or in-transit disease, and primary tumor ulceration status categorize patients with stage III disease.
- For stage IV disease, location of distant metastases (skin/subcutaneous/nodal vs lung vs nonlung visceral) and increased lactate dehydrogenase levels categorize patients with M1 status.
- Other pathologic and clinical factors of the primary tumor have been reported with variable prognostic significance: presence of tumor-infiltrating lymphocytes, absence of regression, younger age, female gender, and extremity location have generally been associated with more favorable outcomes.
- Prognostic factors for sentinel lymph node positivity overlap but are not uniformly congruent with those for survival.

INTRODUCTION

The current (seventh) edition of the American Joint Commission on Cancer (AJCC) staging system for melanoma is now approaching its sixth year since publication and is based on 30,946 patients with stage I, II, and III melanoma and 7972 patients with stage IV melanoma from 17 major medical centers or independent cancer centers.[1] This article reviews the notable changes in the current staging system compared with the last and discusses this in the context of clinical management of patients.

Disclosures: The authors have nothing to disclose.
Department of Surgery, University of Pennsylvania, 3400 Spruce Street, 4 Silverstein, Philadelphia, Pennsylvania 19104, USA
* Corresponding author.
E-mail address: giorgos.karakousis@uphs.upenn.edu

Surg Oncol Clin N Am 24 (2015) 215–227
http://dx.doi.org/10.1016/j.soc.2014.12.001
1055-3207/15/$ – see front matter © 2015 Elsevier Inc. All rights reserved.

Tumor and patient factors are discussed that do not feature in the staging system but that nonetheless carry important prognostic significance.

MELANOMA STAGING SYSTEM

The current AJCC staging system for melanoma is shown in **Tables 1** and **2**.

Stage 0 Melanoma (Melanoma In Situ)

Melanoma in situ refers to a lesion that is not invasive to the dermis. These lesions are thought to have no metastatic potential and as such a carry an excellent prognosis, albeit with some small risk of local recurrence. A surgical excision margin for

Table 1
Seventh edition of the AJCC TNM (tumor, node, metastasis) staging categories for melanoma

T Classification	Thickness (mm)	Additional Stratification
Tis	NA	NA
T1	≤1.00	a: Without ulceration and mitoses <1/mm2 b: With ulceration or mitoses ≥1/mm2
T2	1.01–2.00	a: Without ulceration b: With ulceration
T3	2.01–4.00	a: Without ulceration b: With ulceration
T4	>4.00	a: Without ulceration b: With ulceration
N Classification	**Number of Metastatic Nodes**	**Metastatic Burden**
N0	0	NA
N1	1	a: Micrometastasis (identified on SLN biopsy) b: Macrometastasis (identified on clinical examination)
N2	2–3	a: Micrometastasis (identified on SLN biopsy) b: Macrometastasis (identified on clinical examination) c: In-transit metastases/satellites without nodal metastases
N3	4+ metastatic nodes, matted nodes, or in-transit metastases/satellites with nodal metastases	—
M Classification	**Site**	**Serum LDH Level**
M0	No distant metastases	NA
M1a	Distant skin, subcutaneous, or nodal metastasis	Normal
M1b	Lung metastases	Normal
M1c	All other visceral metastases Any distant metastasis	Normal Increased

Abbreviations: LDH, lactate dehydrogenase; NA, not available; SLN, sentinel lymph node.
   From Edge SB, Byrd DR, Compton CC, editors. AJCC Cancer Staging Manual. 7th edition. New York (NY): Springer, 2010; with permission.

Table 2
Seventh edition of the AJCC stage groupings for melanoma

Clinical Staging	T	N	M
0	Tis	N0	M0
IA	T1a	N0	M0
IB	T1b	N0	M0
	T2a	N0	M0
IIA	T2b	N0	M0
	T3a	N0	M0
IIB	T3b	N0	M0
	T4a	N0	M0
IIC	T4b	N0	M0
III	Any T	N > N0	M0
IV	Any T	Any N	M1
Pathologic Staging			
0	Tis	N0	M0
IA	T1a	N0	M0
IB	T1b	N0	M0
	T2a	N0	M0
IIA	T2b	N0	M0
	T3a	N0	M0
IIB	T3b	N0	M0
	T4a	N0	M0
IIC	T4b	N0	M0
IIIA	T1–4a	N1a	M0
	T1–4a	N2a	M0
IIIB	T1–4b	N1a	M0
	T1–4b	N2a	M0
	T1–4b	N1b	M0
	T1–4a	N2b	M0
	T1–4a	N2c	M0
IIIC	T1–4b	N1b	M0
	T1–4b	N2b	M0
	T1–4b	N2c	M0
	Any T	N3	M0
IV	Any T	Any N	M1

From Edge SB, Byrd DR, Compton CC, editors. AJCC Cancer Staging Manual. 7th edition. New York (NY): Springer, 2010; with permission.

melanoma in situ of 5 mm is considered acceptable by consensus opinion in the current National Comprehensive Cancer Network (NCCN) guidelines.[2]

Stage I and II Melanoma

The 2 primary tumor variables influencing the stage of early localized melanomas that have consistently been shown to be associated with prognosis are tumor thickness (or Breslow depth) and ulceration status.[3–10] For thin melanomas (≤ 1.00 mm or T1), tumor mitotic rate enters as an additional important staging variable in the current staging system, replacing Clark level in the older classification system.[1,11] Thickness is categorically divided for staging purposes (T1, ≤ 1.00 mm; T2, 1.01–2.00 mm; T3, 2.01–4.00; T4, >4.00). The presence of ulceration provides a modification of "b" to the T stage. Nonulcerated melanomas of a particular thickness category are typically grouped together with ulcerated melanomas of the immediately lower thickness category for purposes of stage grouping, except at the 2 extremes of groups, where stage IA includes only T1a lesions and stage IIC includes only T4b lesions. The 10-year survival of patients with T1 melanomas is approximately 92%, compared with only 50% for patients with T4 melanomas.[3] Likewise, ulceration is a strong predictor in patients with melanoma, with 5-year survival rates of 71% for T4a melanomas compared with 53% for T4b melanomas.[3]

Tumor mitotic rate has also been recognized as an important prognostic factor in patients with clinically localized melanoma.[6,12–15] The threshold for defining a lesion as mitogenic is at least 1 mitosis/mm^2 as determined by the hot-spot method.[6,16] When mitotic index is taken into account, Clark level loses its significance in T1 lesions and thus is recommended to be used only if mitotic index information is unavailable for a lesion. The prognostic impact of mitogenicity seems to be greatest in T1 melanomas, for which it is used in the staging system to further risk stratify these lesions.[1] Among nonulcerated T1 melanomas, the 10-year survival rate was 95% in lesions with mitotic rate less than 1/mm^2 compared with 88% for those with mitotic rate greater than or equal to 1/mm^2.[1] Mitotic rate is concordant with tumor thickness, with mean number of mitoses being 1/mm^2 in T1 melanomas compared with 9.6/mm^2 for melanomas greater than 8 mm in depth.[13]

In a multivariate analysis of 10,233 patients with clinically localized (stage I/II) melanoma used in defining the AJCC study cohort, tumor mitotic rate was the second strongest predictor of survival after tumor thickness.[13] However, only approximately 30% of patients received pathologic staging (approximately 40% of the patients had T1 lesions and therefore may not have been recommended for sentinel lymph node (SLN) biopsy), so it is less clear what the impact of mitotic rate would be for deeper lesions when nodal status is known. Another recent study also using the AJCC study cohort suggests that mitotic rate seems to be a strong predictor of survival even among patients with melanoma with microscopic nodal metastases.[17] In this study of more than 1000 stage III patients with nodal micrometastases and mitotic rate data (>90% of whom had undergone an SLN biopsy), tumor mitotic rate was the second most powerful independent predictor of survival after number of nodal metastases.

Stage III Melanoma

Stage III melanoma is defined by the presence of regional metastases in the form of nodal metastases, in-transit disease, or satellitosis (any N disease >0).[1] Determinants of N stage include number of involved lymph nodes, whether there are micrometastases or macrometastases, presence of in-transit disease or satellites, matted nodes, or concomitant nodal disease and in-transit disease or satellitosis. Stage groupings for stage III disease are also affected by the presence of ulceration in the primary tumor (which makes the stage at least IIIB). There is significant heterogeneity in prognosis among stage III patients with survival ranging from 70% 5-year survival for patients with nonulcerated primary melanomas with a single node with micrometastasis to 39% in patients with matted lymph nodes or metastatic lymph nodes with concomitant satellitosis or in-transit disease (N3).[17] It is noteworthy that the presence of melanoma cells in nodal tissue detected by immunohistochemical stains based on melanoma-associated markers and appropriate morphology is sufficient for the establishment of stage III disease.

Among patients with stage III disease, several tumor and patient variables may offer prognosis beyond those incorporated into the staging system, and these variables seem to differ depending on the type of metastasis in the lymph node. In a recent study by Balch and colleagues[17] of 1872 stage III patients with nodal micrometastases, in addition to number of nodal metastases and tumor ulceration status, thickness, age, and anatomic site of the primary were independent predictors of survival. As already noted, when tumor mitotic rate was included in the model, it followed number of nodal metastases as the most significant predictor of survival. Among patients with nodal macrometastases, only patient age was significant in addition to number of tumor-containing nodes and ulceration status of the primary tumor.[17]

Recently, there has been interest in examining the SLN status of the tumor-containing lymph node (ie, SLN or non-SLN) as another prognostic factor for survival. In one study, non-SLN metastatic disease was the most important predictor of survival in patients with stage III disease classified as such by a positive SLN.[18] Even after adjusting for the total number of tumor-bearing nodes, patients with a positive non-SLN showed significantly worse survival than those with SLN-only disease (66 months vs 34 months respectively; $P = .04$).

Other nuances in the prognosis of patients with stage III melanoma may exist that may not be entirely captured by the staging system alone. For example, patients with microsatellitosis are classified as having at least stage IIIB disease. Although microsatellitosis is often concomitantly associated with other negative prognostic features such as tumor ulceration or nodal metastases, in the absence of such features, survival rates may be as high as 90%, comparing favorably with patients with stage IIIB melanoma overall.[19]

Stage IV Disease

Stage IV disease is defined by the presence of distant metastases (M1 disease). M1 disease is further subclassified (in decreasing order of prognosis) into (1) distant skin, subcutaneous or nodal metastases; (2) lung metastases; or (3) other nonlung visceral metastases or any distant metastases with increased lactate dehydrogenase (LDH) level.[1,20] One-year survival rates have historically (before novel immunotherapies and targeted therapies) ranged from 59% for M1a disease to 41% for M1c disease.[11] These statistics have changed and continue to change in the setting of more effective therapies.[21–23] In a recent study of stage IV patients with BRAF V600 mutation, for example, the median survival was 15.9 months and 58% at 12 months, with most of these patients having M1c disease.[24]

OTHER PROGNOSTIC FACTORS FOR SURVIVAL IN PATIENTS WITH MELANOMA

Several other tumor and patient factors have been examined in melanoma but their prognostic significance has been variably reported. There are several possible explanations for this, including that these factors may be less powerful predictors (not captured by smaller sample size studies), variability in pathologic interpretation, and heterogeneity in study populations. A discussion of these pathologic and clinical variables is presented later. These factors are summarized in **Box 1**.

CLINICAL FACTORS
Age

Increasing age is generally associated with decreased disease-specific survival in patients with melanoma. In a recent study of 7756 clinical stage I/II patients using the AJCC database cohort, age greater than 70 years was associated with worse primary tumor characteristics and higher mortality compared with younger patients. Incidence of SLN positivity was lower in this advanced age group.[25] In a related study, increased

---

Box 1
Adverse prognostic features in patients with stage I/II melanoma

Strong: these factors have consistently been found to be independent predictors of survival

Increasing thickness

Present ulceration

Increasing mitotic rate

Weaker: These factors have been found to be predictors of survival but not consistently or independently of other, stronger factors

Increasing age

Male gender

Head and neck anatomic site

Increasing Clark level

Nonsuperficial spreading histology

Present lymphovascular invasion

Present perineural invasion

Present regression

Absent tumor-infiltrating lymphocytes

---

age (along with number of nodal metastases, presence of ulceration, and mitotic index) was independently associated with a worse prognosis among patients with stage III melanoma.[26]

Anatomic Site

Truncal and head and neck anatomic locations for primary melanoma generally are reported to show worse prognoses compared with extremity location. A recent large institutional experience of 2079 patients undergoing SLN biopsy found head and neck melanoma to have the worst disease-free survival compared with other anatomic sites, whereas having the lowest SLN positivity rate.[27] Anatomic location, like age, may carry prognostic significance even in the context of more advanced disease. In a study of stage III patients using the AJCC study cohort, anatomic site (axial compared with extremity) was independently associated with worse survival in patients with micrometastatic nodal disease.[17]

Gender

For reasons that are not well understood, female gender has generally been associated with improved outcomes in patients with melanoma. In a pooled analysis of 4 European Organization for Research and Treatment of Cancer (EORTC) phase III trials with 2672 patients with stage I/II melanoma, female gender was independently associated with more favorable outcomes with respect to time to lymph node and distant metastasis, disease-specific survival, and overall survival.[28] Moreover, this advantage was observed in premenopausal and postmenopausal women. As with more advanced disease, in a pooled analysis of 2734 stage III patients and 1306 stage IV patients from 5 EORTC trials, female gender was associated with improved disease-specific survival compared with male gender.[29] The persistence of the gender effect in advanced disease suggests that biological factors rather than behavioral differences alone account for, at least in part, the variable gender outcomes.

PATHOLOGIC FACTORS OF THE PRIMARY TUMOR
Clark Level

Clark level, a measure of invasion of the tumor through the various skin layers, has historically carried prognostic significance for primary melanoma, with increasing Clark level associated with worse prognosis.[30] Its prognostic significance was perhaps more evident in thin lesions, and as such was included in prior editions of the staging system.[31] More recent reports suggest a lack of significant independent prognostic value for this variable when Breslow depth is considered, and in the current AJCC staging edition, Clark level is replaced by mitotic index (when available) for defining T1b lesions.[1]

Histologic Subtype

There are 4 predominant histologic subtypes of melanoma: superficial spreading (accounting for up to 70% of cases) with prominent radial growth phase; nodular melanoma, characterized by vertical growth phase alone; acral lentiginous, found on palmar and plantar surfaces and subungual locations; and lentigo maligna, which is most commonly seen in the elderly population in sun-exposed areas (particularly the face). Rare subtypes include amelanotic melanoma, which can present challenges in diagnosis, and desmoplastic melanoma (<5%), which tends to have a lower incidence of lymph node metastases but can be associated with higher local recurrence rates.[32] The superficial spreading subtype is generally associated with more favorable prognosis, but, when other stronger prognostic factors (eg, tumor thickness, ulceration) are accounted for, the histologic subtype of the primary tumor does not seem to add significant prognostic value.

Lymphovascular Invasion

Lymphovascular invasion (LVI) has generally been shown to be a strong predictor of regional or SLN metastases. In one study of patients with T2 melanomas, the incidence of SLN positivity was more than 2-fold higher among patients with LVI present compared with LVI absent (25.5% compared with 11.5%).[33] In a study of melanomas from 251 patients with clinical stage I and II disease in the pre-SLN era using an antibody that stains lymphatic endothelium (D2-40), the presence of lymphatic invasion was independently associated with an increased rate of metastases.[34] However, its significance when SLN status is considered is less clear. A recent study that developed a 12-year overall survival nomogram showed LVI to be an independent (albeit weaker) predictor of survival when SLN status was considered in patients with thin melanoma.[35]

Perineural Invasion

Perineural invasion or neurotropism is less commonly noted in pathology reports and less frequently analyzed in prognostic studies and as such has not been frequently associated with melanoma survival outcomes. This variable has been associated with increased rates of local recurrence when present in patients with desmoplastic melanomas.[36]

Regression

Primary tumor regression, characterized by formation of a fibroblastic reaction, has not been shown to carry independent prognostic significance for melanoma-specific survival with any consistency, but has been reported in some studies to be associated with worse survival outcomes, particularly in thin lesions.[37,38] In a recent multicenter trial of 2243 patients with thin melanoma, regression greater than or equal to 50% was identified in 26.3% of the lesions, and was identified as one of the stronger predictors of survival among these patients (hazard ratio, 3.32).[35] Regression may further help to risk stratify patients with thick (T4) melanomas, particularly in the context of known tumor-infiltrating lymphocyte (TIL) status. In one study of T4 melanomas, patients with lesions having absent regression and present TIL showed the most favorable survival outcomes (78% 10-year survival) compared with those with lesions having either absent TIL, present regression, or both (0%–35% 10-year survival).[39] Although its exact significance is unclear, the presence of regression may reflect an ineffectual local immune response to the primary tumor.

Tumor-infiltrating Lymphocytes

The presence of TILs has generally been associated with better survival outcomes, although its prognostic significance has also been inconsistently reported. In one of the early prognostic models for clinical stage I cutaneous melanoma by Clark and colleagues,[6] TIL was identified as an important predictor of survival. In a more recent study of 3330 invasive melanomas from the Genes, Environment, and Melanoma (GEM) study, the presence of nonbrisk TIL grade and brisk TIL grade were associated with a 30% and 50% decrease in melanoma-related death compared with absent TIL after adjustment for AJCC tumor stage, age, gender, and anatomic site.[40] The inconsistent reporting for the prognostic significance of TIL may be a function of heterogeneity in primary tumor thickness considered in the studies (with TIL prognostic significance seeming to be greater in thicker lesions or at least with vertical growth phase), the variability of pathologic grading of TIL, and the issue of whether TIL may be an important predictor of SLN status, but becomes a less significant predictor of survival when the SLN status is known.[41–45]

MOLECULAR AND SERUM FACTORS

Clinicopathologic factors currently form the basis for most clinical care. Despite the identification of the numerous factors described earlier, there remains a wide heterogeneity of survival within individual stages. As such, recent research has focused on molecular biomarkers in an effort to improve prognostication. Several genetic mutations have now been associated with prognosis including ERBB3, AKT, MITF, PTEN, BCL2, and NCOA3.[46–50] However, the relative prognostic value of genetic variants after adjustment for the traditional clinicopathologic variables, particularly nodal status and Breslow depth, are not well studied. Testing for genetic variants has therefore not been routinely incorporated into clinical practice.

The 1 serum marker that has been fully accepted for its prognostic value is LDH. LDH level has long been recognized as being increased in the serum of patients with melanoma.[51] It was recently associated with poor survival and, in patients with advanced melanoma, was the only such tumor marker in a multivariate analysis to be significantly associated with outcome.[52,53] These findings led to the incorporation of LDH into the staging criteria for patients with metastatic disease.[1]

With the development of effective targeted agents, particular interest has recently focused on the prognostic value of the BRAF mutation.[54] A surprising paucity of data exists on this topic. A recent study by Long and colleagues[55] suggests that an activating mutation in BRAF is associated with a poorer prognosis than wild-type BRAF, although treatment with BRAF-targeted therapy may abrogate the detrimental effects of the mutation. A second study that included both BRAF and NRAS mutations in the analysis found that NRAS but not BRAF mutations were associated with decreased overall survival in a multivariate analysis.[56] As the ability to screen for numerous mutations simultaneously becomes more readily available, the interaction among various mutations, as well as the relative contributions to prognosis that these mutations add to the traditional clinicopathologic factors, will likely be an active area of study. To date, there is no definite role for genetic testing in order to obtain prognostic information.

PROGNOSTIC FACTORS FOR SENTINEL LYMPH NODE AND NON–SENTINEL LYMPH NODE POSITIVITY

SLN status has been identified as the single strongest predictor of survival in patients with clinically localized melanoma. The Multicenter Selective Lymphadenectomy Trial 1 (MSLT-1) confirmed the prognostic value of SLN biopsy in patients with melanoma of 1.2 to 3.5 mm thickness.[57] Multiple retrospective studies have now corroborated this finding in patients with thin and thick melanomas.[58–63]

Because of its prognostic importance, SLN biopsy is recommended for all patients with melanoma greater than 1 mm in thickness.[2] In patients with thin melanoma, the overall rate of SLN positivity is approximately 5%, which has led to significant debate regarding the appropriate indications for the procedure in these patients. Numerous studies have sought to define the predictors of SLN positivity in patients with thin melanoma in order to select patients for the procedure. These studies have variably identified several factors, including age, sex, Clark level, thickness, the presence of vertical growth phase, mitotic rate, ulceration, and LVI, as being associated with SLN positivity.[59,61,64–71]

Current NCCN guidelines incorporate thickness as the primary predictor of SLN metastasis in thin melanoma. In patients with primary lesions 0.76 to 1.00 mm in thickness, SLN biopsy should be considered, and it should be recommended in these patients if the lesion is mitogenic or ulceration is present (T1b lesions $\geq$0.76 mm). In patients with melanomas less than 0.76 mm thick, SLN biopsy is not routinely recommended but may be considered if high-risk features (mitoses, ulceration, LVI) are present.[2] In some of the largest and most recent series investigating predictors of SLN positivity in patients with thin melanoma, Clark level has been independently predictive of nodal positivity, whereas some other tumor factors present in the staging system were not consistently independently prognostic.[65,67] These studies highlight the concept that factors associated with nodal metastasis are not always congruent with those associated with survival.

SUMMARY

The current AJCC system for melanoma incorporates thickness, ulceration, and mitotic index as primary tumor factors that define patients with stage I and II disease. Number and size (micro vs macro) of nodal metastases, presence of satellitosis and in-transit disease, and tumor ulceration status categorize patients with stage III disease. Presence and location of distant metastatic disease (skin/soft tissue/nodal, lung, or other nonvisceral) and increased LDH level define and prognosticate patients with stage IV disease. Several other pathologic factors (TIL, LVI, perineural invasion, regression, Clark level) and clinical variables (age, gender, and anatomic site) have been studied with variable prognostic significance. Various molecular markers have recently been investigated for their prognostic significance, although sufficient data are currently lacking to support their use in clinical care. Prognostic factors for SLN positivity beyond tumor thickness are also an area of active study, particularly in patients with T1 melanomas; these factors are not always congruent with those predictive of survival.

REFERENCES

1. Balch CM, Gershenwald JE, Soong SJ, et al. Final version of 2009 AJCC melanoma staging and classification. J Clin Oncol 2009;27:6199–206.
2. Coit DG, Andtbacka R, Anker CJ, et al. Melanoma. J Natl Compr Canc Netw 2012;10:366–400.
3. Balch CM, Soong SJ, Gershenwald JE, et al. Prognostic factors analysis of 17,600 melanoma patients: validation of the American Joint Committee on Cancer melanoma staging system. J Clin Oncol 2001;19:3622–34.
4. Breslow A. Thickness, cross-sectional areas and depth of invasion in the prognosis of cutaneous melanoma. Ann Surg 1970;172:902–8.
5. Barnhill RL, Fine JA, Roush GC, et al. Predicting five-year outcome for patients with cutaneous melanoma in a population-based study. Cancer 1996;78:427–32.
6. Clark WH Jr, Elder DE, Guerry D, et al. Model predicting survival in stage I melanoma based on tumor progression. J Natl Cancer Inst 1989;81:1893–904.
7. Balch CM, Soong S, Ross MI, et al. Long-term results of a multi-institutional randomized trial comparing prognostic factors and surgical results for intermediate thickness melanomas (1.0 to 4.0 mm). Intergroup Melanoma Surgical Trial. Ann Surg Oncol 2000;7:87–97.
8. Retsas S, Henry K, Mohammed MQ, et al. Prognostic factors of cutaneous melanoma and a new staging system proposed by the American Joint Committee on Cancer (AJCC): validation in a cohort of 1284 patients. Eur J Cancer 2002;38:511–6.
9. Balch CM, Wilkerson JA, Murad TM, et al. The prognostic significance of ulceration of cutaneous melanoma. Cancer 1980;45:3012–7.
10. Kim SH, Garcia C, Rodriguez J, et al. Prognosis of thick cutaneous melanoma. J Am Coll Surg 1999;188:241–7.
11. Balch CM, Buzaid AC, Soong SJ, et al. Final version of the American Joint Committee on Cancer staging system for cutaneous melanoma. J Clin Oncol 2001;19:3635–48.
12. Azzola MF, Shaw HM, Thompson JF, et al. Tumor mitotic rate is a more powerful prognostic indicator than ulceration in patients with primary cutaneous melanoma: an analysis of 3661 patients from a single center. Cancer 2003;97:1488–98.
13. Thompson JF, Soong SJ, Balch CM, et al. Prognostic significance of mitotic rate in localized primary cutaneous melanoma: an analysis of patients in the multi-institutional American Joint Committee on Cancer melanoma staging database. J Clin Oncol 2011;29:2199–205.
14. Francken AB, Shaw HM, Thompson JF, et al. The prognostic importance of tumor mitotic rate confirmed in 1317 patients with primary cutaneous melanoma and long follow-up. Ann Surg Oncol 2004;11:426–33.
15. Gimotty PA, Guerry D, Ming ME, et al. Thin primary cutaneous malignant melanoma: a prognostic tree for 10-year metastasis is more accurate than American Joint Committee on Cancer staging. J Clin Oncol 2004;22:3668–76.
16. Scolyer RA, Shaw HM, Thompson JF, et al. Interobserver reproducibility of histopathologic prognostic variables in primary cutaneous melanomas. Am J Surg Pathol 2003;27:1571–6.
17. Balch CM, Gershenwald JE, Soong SJ, et al. Multivariate analysis of prognostic factors among 2,313 patients with stage III melanoma: comparison of nodal micrometastases versus macrometastases. J Clin Oncol 2010;28:2452–9.
18. Pasquali S, Mocellin S, Mozzillo N, et al. Nonsentinel lymph node status in patients with cutaneous melanoma: results from a multi-institution prognostic study. J Clin Oncol 2014;32:935–41.

19. Bartlett EK, Gupta M, Datta J, et al. Prognosis of patients with melanoma and microsatellitosis undergoing sentinel lymph node biopsy. Ann Surg Oncol 2014; 21:1016–23.
20. Barth A, Wanek LA, Morton DL. Prognostic factors in 1,521 melanoma patients with distant metastases. J Am Coll Surg 1995;181:193–201.
21. Chapman PB, Hauschild A, Robert C, et al. Improved survival with vemurafenib in melanoma with BRAF V600E mutation. N Engl J Med 2011;364:2507–16.
22. Hodi FS, O'Day SJ, McDermott DF, et al. Improved survival with ipilimumab in patients with metastatic melanoma. N Engl J Med 2010;363:711–23.
23. Wolchok JD, Kluger H, Callahan MK, et al. Nivolumab plus ipilimumab in advanced melanoma. N Engl J Med 2013;369:122–33.
24. Sosman JA, Kim KB, Schuchter L, et al. Survival in BRAF V600-mutant advanced melanoma treated with vemurafenib. N Engl J Med 2012;366:707–14.
25. Balch CM, Thompson JF, Gershenwald JE, et al. Age as a predictor of sentinel node metastasis among patients with localized melanoma: an inverse correlation of melanoma mortality and incidence of sentinel node metastasis among young and old patients. Ann Surg Oncol 2014;21:1075–81.
26. Balch CM, Soong SJ, Gershenwald JE, et al. Age as a prognostic factor in patients with localized melanoma and regional metastases. Ann Surg Oncol 2013;20:3961–8.
27. Fadaki N, Li R, Parrett B, et al. Is head and neck melanoma different from trunk and extremity melanomas with respect to sentinel lymph node status and clinical outcome? Ann Surg Oncol 2013;20:3089–97.
28. Joosse A, Collette S, Suciu S, et al. Superior outcome of women with stage I/II cutaneous melanoma: pooled analysis of four European Organisation for Research and Treatment of Cancer phase III trials. J Clin Oncol 2012;30:2240–7.
29. Joosse A, Collette S, Suciu S, et al. Sex is an independent prognostic indicator for survival and relapse/progression-free survival in metastasized stage III to IV melanoma: a pooled analysis of five European Organisation for Research and Treatment of Cancer randomized controlled trials. J Clin Oncol 2013;31: 2337–46.
30. Clark WH Jr, From L, Bernardino EA, et al. The histogenesis and biologic behavior of primary human malignant melanomas of the skin. Cancer Res 1969;29:705–27.
31. Pontikes LA, Temple WJ, Cassar SL, et al. Influence of level and depth on recurrence rate in thin melanomas. Am J Surg 1993;165:225–8.
32. Murali R, Shaw HM, Lai K, et al. Prognostic factors in cutaneous desmoplastic melanoma: a study of 252 patients. Cancer 2010;116:4130–8.
33. Mays MP, Martin RC, Burton A, et al. Should all patients with melanoma between 1 and 2 mm Breslow thickness undergo sentinel lymph node biopsy? Cancer 2010;116:1535–44.
34. Xu X, Chen L, Guerry D, et al. Lymphatic invasion is independently prognostic of metastasis in primary cutaneous melanoma. Clin Cancer Res 2012;18:229–37.
35. Maurichi A, Miceli R, Camerini T, et al. Prediction of survival in patients with thin melanoma: results from a multi-institution study. J Clin Oncol 2014;32: 2479–85.
36. Quinn MJ, Crotty KA, Thompson JF, et al. Desmoplastic and desmoplastic neurotropic melanoma: experience with 280 patients. Cancer 1998;83:1128–35.
37. Ronan SG, Eng AM, Briele HA, et al. Thin malignant melanomas with regression and metastases. Arch Dermatol 1987;123:1326–30.
38. Slingluff CL Jr, Vollmer RT, Reintgen DS, et al. Lethal "thin" malignant melanoma. Identifying patients at risk. Ann Surg 1988;208:150–61.

39. Cintolo JA, Gimotty P, Blair A, et al. Local immune response predicts survival in patients with thick (t4) melanomas. Ann Surg Oncol 2013;20:3610–7.
40. Thomas NE, Busam KJ, From L, et al. Tumor-infiltrating lymphocyte grade in primary melanomas is independently associated with melanoma-specific survival in the population-based genes, environment and melanoma study. J Clin Oncol 2013;31:4252–9.
41. Taylor RC, Patel A, Panageas KS, et al. Tumor-infiltrating lymphocytes predict sentinel lymph node positivity in patients with cutaneous melanoma. J Clin Oncol 2007;25:869–75.
42. Clemente CG, Mihm MC Jr, Bufalino R, et al. Prognostic value of tumor infiltrating lymphocytes in the vertical growth phase of primary cutaneous melanoma. Cancer 1996;77:1303–10.
43. Day CL Jr, Lew RA, Mihm MC Jr, et al. A multivariate analysis of prognostic factors for melanoma patients with lesions greater than or equal to 3.65 mm in thickness. The importance of revealing alternative Cox models. Ann Surg 1982;195:44–9.
44. Elder DE, Guerry D, VanHorn M, et al. The role of lymph node dissection for clinical stage I malignant melanoma of intermediate thickness (1.51–3.99 mm). Cancer 1985;56:413–8.
45. Tuthill RJ, Unger JM, Liu PY, et al. Risk assessment in localized primary cutaneous melanoma: a Southwest Oncology Group study evaluating nine factors and a test of the Clark logistic regression prediction model. Am J Clin Pathol 2002;118:504–11.
46. Dai DL, Martinka M, Li G. Prognostic significance of activated Akt expression in melanoma: a clinicopathologic study of 292 cases. J Clin Oncol 2005;23: 1473–82.
47. Fecker LF, Geilen CC, Tchernev G, et al. Loss of proapoptotic Bcl-2-related multidomain proteins in primary melanomas is associated with poor prognosis. J Invest Dermatol 2006;126:1366–71.
48. Mikhail M, Velazquez E, Shapiro R, et al. PTEN expression in melanoma: relationship with patient survival, Bcl-2 expression, and proliferation. Clin Cancer Res 2005;11:5153–7.
49. Rangel J, Torabian S, Shaikh L, et al. Prognostic significance of nuclear receptor coactivator-3 overexpression in primary cutaneous melanoma. J Clin Oncol 2006; 24:4565–9.
50. Salti GI, Manougian T, Farolan M, et al. Micropthalmia transcription factor: a new prognostic marker in intermediate-thickness cutaneous malignant melanoma. Cancer Res 2000;60:5012–6.
51. Hill BR, Levi C. Elevation of a serum component in neoplastic disease. Cancer Res 1954;14:513–5.
52. Campora E, Repetto L, Giuntini P, et al. LDH in the follow-up of stage I malignant melanoma. Eur J Cancer Clin Oncol 1988;24:277–8.
53. Deichmann M, Benner A, Bock M, et al. S100-Beta, melanoma-inhibiting activity, and lactate dehydrogenase discriminate progressive from nonprogressive American Joint Committee on Cancer stage IV melanoma. J Clin Oncol 1999;17:1891–6.
54. Flaherty KT. Is it good or bad to find a BRAF mutation? J Clin Oncol 2011;29: 1229–30.
55. Long GV, Menzies AM, Nagrial AM, et al. Prognostic and clinicopathologic associations of oncogenic BRAF in metastatic melanoma. J Clin Oncol 2011;29: 1239–46.
56. Jakob JA, Bassett RL Jr, Ng CS, et al. NRAS mutation status is an independent prognostic factor in metastatic melanoma. Cancer 2012;118:4014–23.

57. Morton DL, Thompson JF, Cochran AJ, et al. Sentinel-node biopsy or nodal observation in melanoma. N Engl J Med 2006;355:1307–17.
58. Karakousis GC, Gimotty PA, Czerniecki BJ, et al. Regional nodal metastatic disease is the strongest predictor of survival in patients with thin vertical growth phase melanomas: a case for SLN staging biopsy in these patients. Ann Surg Oncol 2007;14:1596–603.
59. Murali R, Haydu LE, Quinn MJ, et al. Sentinel lymph node biopsy in patients with thin primary cutaneous melanoma. Ann Surg 2012;255:128–33.
60. Warycha MA, Zakrzewski J, Ni Q, et al. Meta-analysis of sentinel lymph node positivity in thin melanoma (<or = 1 mm). Cancer 2009;115:869–79.
61. Wright BE, Scheri RP, Ye X, et al. Importance of sentinel lymph node biopsy in patients with thin melanoma. Arch Surg 2008;143:892–9 [discussion: 899–900].
62. Mozzillo N, Pennacchioli E, Gandini S, et al. Sentinel node biopsy in thin and thick melanoma. Ann Surg Oncol 2013;20:2780–6.
63. Scoggins CR, Bowen AL, Martin RC 2nd, et al. Prognostic information from sentinel lymph node biopsy in patients with thick melanoma. Arch Surg 2010; 145:622–7.
64. Kesmodel SB, Karakousis GC, Botbyl JD, et al. Mitotic rate as a predictor of sentinel lymph node positivity in patients with thin melanomas. Ann Surg Oncol 2005;12:449–58.
65. Bartlett EK, Gimotty PA, Sinnamon AJ, et al. Clark level risk stratifies patients with mitogenic thin melanomas for sentinel lymph node biopsy. Ann Surg Oncol 2014; 21:643–9.
66. Cecchi R, Buralli L, Innocenti S, et al. Sentinel lymph node biopsy in patients with thin melanomas. J Dermatol 2007;34:512–5.
67. Han D, Zager JS, Shyr Y, et al. Clinicopathologic predictors of sentinel lymph node metastasis in thin melanoma. J Clin Oncol 2013;31:4387–93.
68. Kunte C, Geimer T, Baumert J, et al. Prognostic factors associated with sentinel lymph node positivity and effect of sentinel status on survival: an analysis of 1049 patients with cutaneous melanoma. Melanoma Res 2010;20:330–7.
69. Lowe JB, Hurst E, Moley JF, et al. Sentinel lymph node biopsy in patients with thin melanoma. Arch Dermatol 2003;139:617–21.
70. Oliveira Filho RS, Ferreira LM, Biasi LJ, et al. Vertical growth phase and positive sentinel node in thin melanoma. Braz J Med Biol Res 2003;36:347–50.
71. Ranieri JM, Wagner JD, Wenck S, et al. The prognostic importance of sentinel lymph node biopsy in thin melanoma. Ann Surg Oncol 2006;13:927–32.

Pathology of Melanoma

David E. Elder, MB ChB, FRCPA

KEYWORDS

- Melanoma • Classification • Diagnosis • Prognosis • Histopathology

KEY POINTS

- Pathologic evaluation of a clinically selected lesion remains the "gold standard" for diagnosis of melanoma.
- Ancillary diagnostic techniques are becoming available that may enhance the specificity of pathologic diagnosis.
- Pathologic attributes are important for predicting outcome and planning therapy.

DEFINITION AND DIAGNOSIS OF MELANOMA

Malignant melanoma may be simply defined as a malignant neoplasm derived from melanocytes. Most melanocytes reside in the skin in the basal layer of the epidermis, separated by keratinocytes.[1] Other sites where melanocytes may exist and melanomas may occur include the uveal tract of the eye and various mucosal surfaces, such as the sinonasal mucosa, oral mucosa, and vulva.

Reproducibility of diagnosis of melanocytic proliferations is good for wholly benign lesions such as compound nevi, and for fully malignant lesions such as American Joint Committee on Cancer (AJCC) stage 2 melanomas. Distinctions among various patterns of atypical nevi, melanoma in situ, and "thin" invasive melanomas are less reliable. There is also considerable variation of terminology from institution to institution. In a recent proposal that might alleviate some problems of uncertainty in classification, it has been suggested that lesions might be placed into treatment categories termed "MPath-Dx," analogous to a similar scheme used for codification of mammograms. In this system, the usual terms for a particular institution would be employed for diagnosis and an MPath-Dx category, delineating possible considerations for management would be appended, with the goals of facilitating communication among institutions and of enabling studies of outcome in relation to management of homogeneous categories of melanocytic proliferations.[2]

The author has nothing to disclose.
Department of Pathology and Laboratory Medicine, Hospital of the University of Pennsylvania, 3400 Spruce Street, Philadelphia, PA 19104, USA
E-mail address: David.Elder@uphs.upenn.edu

Surg Oncol Clin N Am 24 (2015) 229–237
http://dx.doi.org/10.1016/j.soc.2014.12.002
1055-3207/15/$ – see front matter © 2015 Elsevier Inc. All rights reserved.

CLASSIFICATION AND HISTOPATHOLOGIC DIAGNOSIS OF MELANOMA

Although it has been suggested that melanoma is 1 disease, it is not true that 1 set of criteria can be used to diagnose all cases of melanoma. To the contrary, there is striking variation among different forms of melanoma, which has led to their being categorized in various classification schemes. An important foundation of classification of melanomas is based on patterns of evolution of melanoma, from a patch or plaque in the skin termed the "radial growth phase" (RGP), to a tumorigenic proliferation called the "vertical growth phase" (VGP), with increasing risk of metastasis. In the current World Health Organization classification, melanomas are classified mainly on the basis of their RGP components into superficial spreading, lentigo maligna, and acral subtypes. Tumors that lack an RGP are termed "nodular melanoma."[3] This category accounts for only about 10% of melanomas but a disproportionate number of deaths, because all of them are in the VGP (**Box 1**).[4]

RADIAL GROWTH PHASE: NONTUMORIGENIC MELANOMA

Most melanomas begin as a patch or plaque in the skin that spreads along the radii of an increasingly irregular circle in the skin, and is therefore known as the RGP, a term derived from clinical morphology but more often applied histologically. Clinically, the lesions tend to acquire attributes that have been captured in a number of algorithms,[5] the best known of which is the "A, B, C, D, E" rule, in which A stands for asymmetry, B for border irregularity, C for color variegation, D for diameter greater than 4 mm, and E variously stands for "evolution" or "elevation." This clinical morphology is, of course, the gross pathology of the melanoma.

  Histologically, there is an increased number of cytologically atypical melanocytes in the epidermis. These lose the normal contact inhibition, which leads to the separation of their cell bodies by keratinocytes. There are 2 important patterns of proliferation. The best known of these is that of nests or clusters of melanocytes, which tend to rise up into the epidermis, partially replacing it in what has been termed a "buckshot scatter" or "pagetoid" pattern, the latter term reflecting a histologic resemblance to Paget's disease of the breast (**Fig. 1**). The other main pattern of proliferation is that

---

Box 1
World Health Organization classification of malignant melanoma

Superficial spreading melanoma

Nodular melanoma

Lentigo maligna

Acral–lentiginous melanoma

Desmoplastic melanoma

Melanoma arising from blue nevus

Melanoma arising in a giant congenital nevus

Melanoma of childhood

Nevoid melanoma

Persistent melanoma

Adapted from LeBoit P, Burg G, Weedon D, et al. Melanocytic tumors. In: LeBoit PE, Burg G, Weedon D, et al. Pathology and genetics of skin tumors. Lyon (France): IARC Press; 2006. p. 50; with permission.

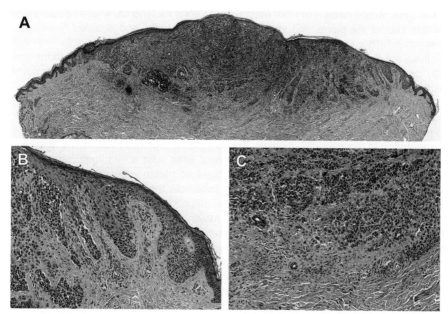

Fig. 1. (*A*) Malignant melanoma. There is a bulky vertical growth phase (VGP) in the center, extending to a depth of 1.4 mm, with adjacent radial growth phase (RGP) in the epidermis on each side. (*B*) Pagetoid scatter of atypical cells into the epidermis at right; atypical cells of the VGP infiltrating the dermis at the left. (*C*) Atypical VGP cells above a remnant of a dermal nevus at the base of the lesion. Hematoxylin and eosin stains. Original magnifications 2×, 10×, 20×.

of continuous basal proliferation, where the atypical melanocytes replace basal keratinocytes. This pattern is termed "lentiginous" because it resembles the pattern of proliferation of melanocytes in lentigines. In lentiginous proliferations, single cells tend to predominate over nests. These patterns have been well illustrated in a recent study that correlated phenotypic features with mutation status of the oncogenes BRAF or NRAS. Melanomas with BRAF mutations showed distinct morphologic features such as increased nest formation and pagetoid scatter, thickening of the involved epidermis, and sharper demarcation to the surrounding skin; they had larger, rounder, and more pigmented tumor cells. These were also associated with a lesser degree of chronic solar damage (CSD), and generally corresponded to the superficial spreading melanoma subtype. The NRAS or other oncogene-related melanomas tended to have a predominantly lentiginous pattern, with few nests, less pigment, smaller cells, and a higher degree of CSD, corresponding to the lentigo maligna subtype.[6]

The patterns of proliferation in the epidermis—nested, pagetoid, or lentiginous—correlate with clinical and epidemiologic evidence that have long been known and have been formulated recently in terms of a "divergent pathways hypothesis."[7] In this hypothesis, there are 2 major patterns of sun exposure that correlate with melanoma risk. In one of these patterns, "acute–intermittent" sun exposure (eg, weekend/recreational activity) results in melanomas that tend to occur in a younger age group and in skin with mild to moderate CSD. These melanomas histologically tend to exhibit features of the "BRAF/superficial spreading melanoma" subtypes. In the other pattern, "chronic–continuous" sun exposure that can result from occupational exposure tends to be associated with melanomas with features more characteristic of lentigo maligna melanoma, and associated with moderate to severe CSD.

The other major pattern of RGP melanoma is acral melanoma, which occurs in the hairless skin of the palms and soles, and also in the nails, and is called "subungual melanoma." This form of melanoma is not likely to be caused by solar damage because the thick stratum corneum in acral sites diffuses sunlight and sunburn typically does not occur, even after prolonged exposure. These melanomas bear some resemblance to lentigo maligna melanoma in that the predominant pattern of growth is lentiginous, which has resulted in their being characterized as "acral–lentiginous melanoma." There are other histologic differences between acral–lentiginous melanoma and lentigo maligna melanoma, including larger cell size and more prominent pigmentation in the majority of cases. These acral–lentiginous melanomas also tend to resemble melanomas occurring in mucosal sites with a histologic pattern that has been termed "mucosal–lentiginous." Pagetoid melanomas also occur in acral sites and their genomic biology is said to resemble those of the lentiginous acral melanomas, so that the preferred current classification is "acral melanoma."[3]

In terms of AJCC staging criteria, the vast majority of RGP melanomas are "thin" by Breslow's criteria, and by Clark's levels of invasion the majority of them fall into levels I (in situ) and II (invasive into the papillary dermis but failing to fill and expand it and therefore in most cases nontumorigenic and associated with an excellent prognosis).[8] In a study by Gimotty and colleagues[9] of more than 26,000 melanoma cases from the Surveillance, Epidemiology, and End Results tumor registry, a subset of almost 50% of the cases had a probability of 10-year survival of 99% based on the properties of ulceration, mitogenicity, Clark's levels, Breslow thickness of less than 0.78 mm, and age less than 60 years. Most of these cases represent "pure" RGP cases.

VERTICAL GROWTH PHASE: TUMORIGENIC MELANOMA

After a variable period of evolution of the RGP, these lesions are at risk of acquiring the next stage of progression, called VGP, in which the lesional cells may grow up above the level of the skin, or invade down into the skin, forming a tumorigenic or mass lesion developing within the antecedent plaque (see **Fig. 1**) or in some cases apparently de novo. Nodular melanoma is a pattern of melanoma in which a tumorigenic VGP is formed and in which an antecedent RGP component is not evident.[10] There may have been a short lived, in situ component that was overwhelmed by a tumorigenic VGP. Nodular melanomas therefore lack the clinical "ABCDE" criteria and also lack many of the histologic features mentioned, such as pagetoid scatter and lentiginous proliferation.

The VGP results in most of the attributes of melanoma that account for risk of metastasis and death. These include tumor thickness according to Breslow; Clark's level of invasion, which is a measure of extension into the skin; the mitotic rate; the presence or absence of ulceration, which is almost always associated with the VGP rather than the RGP; and other attributes considered to be of lesser importance such as tumor infiltrating lymphocytes, RGP regression, lymphovascular invasion, and others.

An important VGP variant is *desmoplastic melanoma* (DM). This condition may be difficult to diagnose both histologically and clinically, and if tumor is left on the margin it will usually recur, often as a more significant lesion. It has been recognized that "pure" DM has a better prognosis than its microstaging attributes might suggest; however, when DM is "mixed" with a component of epithelioid growth, the prognosis is significantly worse.[11] Sentinel node involvement is less likely to occur with "pure" DM; however, opinions about the utility of sentinel node biopsy are mixed.[12] Neurotropism is relatively more common in DM and increases the risk of local recurrence in any melanoma.[13]

IMMUNOHISTOCHEMICAL MARKERS FOR MELANOMA DIAGNOSIS AND PROGNOSIS

Immunohistochemical markers can be divided into 2 major categories. In the first, which can be termed "differentiation markers," immunohistochemistry is used to distinguish melanomas from simulants. These in turn can be divided into simulants of the RGP and VGP. Examples of simulants of pagetoid melanoma include Paget's disease itself, pagetoid lymphoproliferative conditions, and pagetoid squamous cell carcinoma. Examples of simulants of VGP melanoma include poorly differentiated epithelioid and/or spindle cell malignancies. Reliable markers for melanocytic differentiation include several antigens related to the pigmentary apparatus including HMB 45, Melan-A/Mart, and tyrosinase. Other markers include transcription factors and other regulatory proteins such as MITF and Sox 10, which are nuclear markers that may provide a more crisp definition of cell types in some circumstances.

These differentiation markers can also be used to highlight patterns of proliferation, such as pagetoid scatter or continuous basal proliferation, that are of importance in making the diagnosis and may be obscured for example by an inflammatory component. Thus, Melan-A/Mart and MITF or Sox10 are often used in superficial atypical melanocytic proliferations where the differential diagnosis lies between an atypical nevus and a subtle melanoma.[14,15]

In a very limited category of immunohistochemistry stains that may be termed "progression markers" are markers that may be used to support a malignant versus a benign diagnosis, or to assess degrees of malignancy. Immunostains in this category include HMB 45, which can be used as a differentiation marker, highlighting cells near the surface of benign lesions in a top heavy pattern, and staining melanomas in a more homogeneous manner. The proliferation marker Ki-67, which labels cells in cycle, can be used to assess proliferation, which is helpful for diagnosis in some cases. Staining for p16 can be used as a shortcut to ruling out homozygous 9P21 loss, which is associated with malignancy as discussed elsewhere in this article. Although these markers may have some utility in practice as adjunct diagnostic tests, a recent, extensive meta-analysis of the existing data concluded that no molecular prognostic biomarker has yet been translated into clinical practice, and that conventional tissue biomarkers, such as Breslow thickness, ulceration, mitotic rate, and lymph node positivity, remain the backbone prognostic indicators in melanoma.[16]

GENOMIC MARKERS

Genomic techniques have been developed recently, with the goal of identifying malignant lesions and separating them from benign simulants, such as atypical nevi.[17] Using fluorescence in situ hybridization methodology, loss of chromosome region 9P21 has been associated with aggressive behavior in a small subset of these lesions and represents, arguably, the best evidence-based genomic criterion for identification of lesions with potential competence for metastasis and lethal progression.[18,19] Comparative genomic hybridization methodology can identify similar abnormalities,[20] but has not been studied as rigorously in relation to outcome.

PROGNOSTIC EVALUATION AND AMERICAN JOINT COMMITTEE ON CANCER STAGING

An important part of the pathologic interpretation of melanomas is evaluation of prognosis. Use of AJCC staging criteria is discussed elsewhere in this issue (Chapter 1). Pathologic staging depends on tumor thickness, as first described by Breslow,[21] on the identification of ulceration, and on the identification of dermal mitoses, and also on the identification of metastases (satellites or lymph nodes).

Although studies have demonstrated good reproducibility,[22] each of these can be problematic in certain situations.

Breslow thickness is defined as the depth of the tumor and millimeters from the top of the granular layer of the skin to the deepest invasive tumor cell.[21] Although remarkably robust as a prognostic criterion, Breslow thickness can be influenced by epidermal hyperplasia and by involvement of skin appendages, both of which could lead to a spuriously thicker estimate than might be justified by the biology of the tumor. Such cases can be evaluated descriptively and, in some cases, clinicopathologic correlation might be appropriate to avoid overtreatment.

Ulceration is defined as a loss of continuity of the epidermis with evidence of a host reaction. The latter criterion is applied so that simple loss of the epidermis owing to specimen handling is not interpreted as an ulcer. The diagnosis is reproducible when this definition is used.[23] Although the biology of ulceration is poorly understood, it is a strong marker of poor prognosis in melanoma.

Mitotic rate is defined as the number of mitoses per square millimeter. In the first description of the 2009 AJCC staging system, the mitotic rate variable was defined as "greater than or equal to 1," and this remains the definition.[24] This definition implies that there might be a category of "less than 1." This would be theoretically possible, for example, if a tumor measured 10 mm^2 in area and had 1 mitosis, then the mitotic rate might be interpreted as "0.1". However, studies that identified mitotic rate as an important criterion in melanoma used a "hot spot" method in which the area with the greatest number of mitoses is first identified and then the number of mitoses per square millimeter in that area is counted. In such a system, a tumor with a single mitosis would have a hot spot where the mitotic rate was equal to 1. There are other melanomas in which the area of the invasive component is less than 1 mm^2. One might then consider adjusting the mitotic rate; for example, if 0.5 mm^2 were counted and a single mitosis was found, the mitotic rate might be reported as 2. This could result in some strange results if, for example, 1 mitosis was found in a small nest of, say, 1/10 of a square millimeter in a tiny tumor.

In a clarification of the AJCC staging criteria, Gershenwald and colleagues[25] provided criteria for identification of mitotic rate as follows:

"As detailed in the 7th edition of the AJCC Cancer Staging Manual, the recommended approach to enumerating mitoses is to first find the areas in the dermis containing the most mitotic figures, the so-called hot spot. After counting the mitoses in the hot spot, the count is extended to adjacent fields until an area corresponding to 1 mm^2 is assessed. If no hot spot can be found and mitoses are sparse and randomly scattered throughout the lesion, then a representative mitosis is chosen, and beginning with that field, the count is then extended to adjacent fields until an area corresponding to 1 mm^2 is assessed. The count is then expressed as the number of mitoses/mm^2. To accurately record mitoses, calibration of individual microscopes is recommended; as a guide, 1 mm^2 corresponds to an area corresponding to approximately four high-power fields at 400 × in most, but not all, microscopes. For classifying T1 (i.e., up to and including 1 mm) melanomas, the threshold for a nonulcerated melanoma to be defined as T1b is $\geq$1 mitoses/mm^2. When the invasive component of tumor is <1 mm^2 (in area), the number of mitoses present in 1 mm^2 of dermal tissue that includes the tumor should be enumerated and recorded as a number per square millimeter. Alternatively, in tumors whose invasive component comprises an area of <1 mm^2, the simple presence or absence of a mitosis can be designated as at least 1/mm^2 (i.e., "mitogenic") or 0/mm^2 (i.e., "nonmitogenic"), respectively. At some institutions, when mitotic figures are not found after examining numerous fields, the mitotic count has been described as <1/mm^2. For most tumor registries, the designation "<1/mm^2" is synonymous with zero, as has been customarily used in the past. Although this practice may be continued for historical data, the AJCC Melanoma Staging Committee urges pathologists to use the approach outlined above beginning in 2010."

The property relating to mitoses that is used in the AJCC staging system is "mitogenicity," namely, the presence of even a single mitosis. The presence of mitoses can vary from 1 section plane to another in routine histopathological preparations, and it is recommended that 3 to 5 sections should be studied for the property of mitogenicity. Using a greater number of sections is discouraged because it was not the method used in developing the studies used to support the development of the AJCC model, and also because this practice might unduly consume tissue that might be useful for genomic or other studies.

Microscopic satellites are defined as deposits of tumor that are separated from the main lesion by at least 0.3 mm, and that measure at least 0.05 mm in diameter. When these criteria are used, their diagnosis is reasonably reproducible; however, they are commonly omitted from pathology reports.[22] Clinical satellites are less likely to be problematic, except in a few cases where differentiated epidermotropic metastases can be confused with nevi or with new primary melanomas.[26]

A detailed discussion of *lymph node metastases* is beyond the scope of this article. Issues include the distinction between metastases and capsular nevus cells,[27] the definition and significance of "submicroscopic metastases,"[28] and the definition and significance of extracapsular extension of tumor. In addition, there is considerable interinstitutional variation in the number of sections studied in the examination of sentinel nodes, and in the use of immunohistochemistry.[29,30]

PREDICTIVE MARKERS FOR THERAPY: MOLECULAR TESTING AND SEQUENCING

Pathologic characteristics can also be used to develop predictive markers for therapy. In other tumors such as breast cancer, immunohistochemical studies such as Her2/neu testing are used to predict response to therapy; however, such therapies in general are not available in melanoma. Recently, however, the development of targeted therapy for melanoma has led to a need for molecular testing in the form of sequencing of oncogenes to detect mutations of activating sites.[31] This testing is ideally done in pathology departments because of the need for the strict protocols established in laboratories certified under the Clinical Laboratories Improvement Act (CLIA). Criteria for inspection of laboratories that perform molecular testing have been developed by the College of American Pathologists and other inspecting agencies. Another reason for testing in pathology departments is that these departments are the repositories of the tissue, and pathologic expertise is required to identify the melanoma tissue from surrounding normal tissues for appropriate specificity of testing.

Although there are many methods for sequencing genes, 2 major general categories can be identified, namely traditional sequencing and next-generation sequencing.[32-34] The major difference between these 2 categories is that multiple genes can be sequenced simultaneously by next-generation sequencing and to a greater depth. As discussed elsewhere in this article, histologic properties of melanomas are associated with the underlying mutated oncogenes and these could be used to determine an appropriate order of sequencing. For example, in a patient with metastatic melanoma derived from a lentigo–maligna primary, it might be more appropriate to begin testing for mutated KIT or NRAS rather than for BRAF.[6] BRAF, being the most common mutated oncogene in melanoma overall, is usually the first gene to be tested. By next-generation sequencing, however, multiple genes are sequenced simultaneously. Early results from laboratories that have developed this testing, including our own, confirm that BRAF, NRAS, and KIT are the most commonly mutated oncogenes. However, there is a long "tail of the curve" of oncogenes that are mutated only rarely in melanoma, although perhaps more commonly in other cancers.

A compelling vision for the future is that all tumors will be characterized by their driving oncogenes and perhaps also by suppressor genes and other genomic factors. The success of targeted therapy directed against individual oncogenes, despite its limitations, suggests that a repertoire of targeted agents will be developed that can be used against a variety of different tumors, depending on the results of genetic testing. Nevertheless, it can be predicted that histopathologic diagnosis and surgical therapy will remain mainstays of management for melanoma for the foreseeable future.

REFERENCES

1. Elder DE. Pathological staging of melanoma. Methods Mol Biol 2014;1102: 325–51.
2. Piepkorn MW, Barnhill RL, Elder DE, et al. The MPATH-Dx reporting schema for melanocytic proliferations and melanoma. J Am Acad Dermatol 2014;70:131–41.
3. LeBoit P, Burg G, Weedon D, et al. Melanocytic tumors. In: LeBoit PE, Burg G, Weedon D, et al, editors. Pathology and genetics of skin tumors. Lyon (France): IARC Press; 2006. p. 49–120.
4. Mar V, Roberts H, Wolfe R, et al. Nodular melanoma: a distinct clinical entity and the largest contributor to melanoma deaths in Victoria, Australia. J Am Acad Dermatol 2012;68:568–75.
5. Dolianitis C, Kelly J, Wolfe R, et al. Comparative performance of 4 dermoscopic algorithms by nonexperts for the diagnosis of melanocytic lesions. Arch Dermatol 2005;141:1008–14.
6. Viros A, Fridlyand J, Bauer J, et al. Improving melanoma classification by integrating genetic and morphologic features. PLoS Med 2008;5:e120.
7. Whiteman DC, Watt P, Purdie DM, et al. Melanocytic nevi, solar keratoses, and divergent pathways to cutaneous melanoma. J Natl Cancer Inst 2003;95:806–12.
8. Guerry DI, Synnestvedt M, Elder DE, et al. Lessons from tumor progression: the invasive radial growth phase of melanoma is common, incapable of metastasis, and indolent. J Invest Dermatol 1993;100:342S–5S.
9. Gimotty PA, Elder DE, Fraker DL, et al. Identification of high-risk patients among those diagnosed with thin cutaneous melanomas. J Clin Oncol 2007;25:1129–34.
10. Clark WH Jr, From L, Bernardino EA, et al. The histogenesis and biologic behavior of primary human malignant melanomas of the skin. Cancer Res 1969;29:705–27.
11. Chen LL, Jaimes N, Barker CA, et al. Desmoplastic melanoma: a review. J Am Acad Dermatol 2013;68(5):825–33.
12. Broer PN, Walker ME, Goldberg C, et al. Desmoplastic melanoma: a 12-year experience with sentinel lymph node biopsy. Eur J Surg Oncol 2013;39:681–5.
13. Baer SC, Schultz D, Synnestvedt M, et al. Desmoplasia and neurotropism - prognostic variables in patients with stage I melanoma. Cancer 1995;76:2242–7.
14. Hillesheim PB, Slone S, Kelley D, et al. An immunohistochemical comparison between MiTF and MART-1 with Azure blue counterstaining in the setting of solar lentigo and melanoma in situ. J Cutan Pathol 2011;38(7):565–9.
15. Mohamed A, Gonzalez RS, Lawson D, et al. SOX10 Expression in malignant melanoma, carcinoma, and normal tissues. Appl Immunohistochem Mol Morphol 2012;21:506–10.
16. Mandala M, Massi D. Tissue prognostic biomarkers in primary cutaneous melanoma. Virchows Arch 2014;464:265–81.

17. Busam KJ. Molecular pathology of melanocytic tumors. Semin Diagn Pathol 2013;30:362–74.
18. Gerami P, Cooper C, Bajaj S, et al. Outcomes of atypical spitz tumors with chromosomal copy number aberrations and conventional melanomas in children. Am J Surg Pathol 2013;37:1387–94.
19. Lade-Keller J, Riber-Hansen R, Guldberg P, et al. Immunohistochemical analysis of molecular drivers in melanoma identifies p16 as an independent prognostic biomarker. J Clin Pathol 2014;67:520–8.
20. North JP, Vemula SS, Bastian BC. Chromosomal copy number analysis in melanoma diagnostics. Methods Mol Biol 2014;1102:199–226.
21. Breslow A. Thickness, cross-sectional areas and depth of invasion in the prognosis of cutaneous melanoma. Ann Surg 1970;172:902–8.
22. Niebling MG, Haydu LE, Karim RZ, et al. Reproducibility of AJCC staging parameters in primary cutaneous melanoma: an analysis of 4,924 cases. Ann Surg Oncol 2013;20(12):3969–75.
23. Spatz A, Cook MG, Elder DE, et al. Interobserver reproducibility of ulceration assessment in primary cutaneous melanomas. Eur J Cancer 2003;39:1861–5.
24. Balch CM, Gershenwald JE, Soong SJ, et al. Final version of 2009 AJCC melanoma staging and classification. J Clin Oncol 2009;27:6199–206.
25. Gershenwald JE, Soong SJ, Balch CM. 2010 TNM staging system for cutaneous melanoma and beyond. Ann Surg Oncol 2010;17:1475–7.
26. Bahrami S, Cheng L, Wang M, et al. Clonal relationships between epidermotropic metastatic melanomas and their primary lesions: a loss of heterozygosity and X-chromosome inactivation-based analysis. Mod Pathol 2007;20:821–7.
27. Gambichler T, Scholl L, Stucker M, et al. Clinical characteristics and survival data of melanoma patients with nevus cell aggregates within sentinel lymph nodes. Am J Clin Pathol 2013;139:566–73.
28. van der Ploeg AP, van Akkooi AC, Rutkowski P, et al. Prognosis in patients with sentinel node-positive melanoma is accurately defined by the combined Rotterdam tumor load and Dewar topography criteria. J Clin Oncol 2011;29(16):2206–14.
29. Cole CM, Ferringer T. Histopathologic evaluation of the sentinel lymph node for malignant melanoma: the unstandardized process. Am J Dermatopathol 2014;36(1):80–7.
30. Dekker J, Duncan LM. Lack of standards for the detection of melanoma in sentinel lymph nodes: a survey and recommendations. Arch Pathol Lab Med 2013;137:1603–9.
31. Heim D, Budczies J, Stenzinger A, et al. Cancer beyond organ and tissue specificity: next-generation-sequencing gene mutation data reveal complex genetic similarities across major cancers. Int J Cancer 2014;135(10):2362–9.
32. Pritchard CC, Salipante SJ, Koehler K, et al. Validation and implementation of targeted capture and sequencing for the detection of actionable mutation, copy number variation, and gene rearrangement in clinical cancer specimens. J Mol Diagn 2014;16:56–67.
33. Lade-Keller J, Romer KM, Guldberg P, et al. Evaluation of BRAF mutation testing methodologies in formalin-fixed, paraffin-embedded cutaneous melanomas. J Mol Diagn 2013;15:70–80.
34. Lopez-Rios F, Angulo B, Gomez B, et al. Comparison of testing methods for the detection of BRAF V600E mutations in malignant melanoma: pre-approval validation study of the companion diagnostic test for vemurafenib. PLoS One 2013;8: e53733.

Surgical Management of Primary and Recurrent Melanoma

Jeffrey M. Farma, MD[a],*, Nandini Kulkarni, MD[a], Cary Hsu, MD[b,c]

KEYWORDS

- Melanoma • Biopsy technique • Excision • Local recurrence

KEY POINTS

- Early diagnosis of melanoma improves prognosis.
- Optimal margin width depends on the stage of the primary.
- Surgical excision is the preferred treatment of recurrent melanoma.

INTRODUCTION

Melanoma accounts for less than 2% of skin cancer cases, but is responsible for most skin cancer–related deaths. It is estimated that there will be 76,100 new diagnoses of melanoma and 9710 deaths in the United States in 2014.[1]

Surgery continues to be the mainstay of care in the management of melanoma, whether it is for diagnostic, therapeutic, or palliative purposes. Forty years ago, most melanomas were excised widely with 3- to 5-cm margins, and many centers treated regional lymph nodes with routine elective lymph node dissection. This was based on the observation of local and locoregional recurrence in cases where the melanoma was narrowly excised, and it was found that surgical treatment of recurrence was difficult to impossible.[2]

In some centers, wide excision of the primary melanoma was performed in continuity with excision of a broad strip of skin, subcutaneous tissue, and the nearest anatomic group of lymph nodes. This was based on Hogarth Pringle's advice from three cases that he published in 1908.[3,4] Over the past 40 years, there has been dramatic change in

The authors have nothing to disclose.
[a] Department of Surgical Oncology, Fox Chase Cancer Center, 333 Cottman Avenue, Philadelphia, PA 19111, USA; [b] Division of General Surgery, Department of Surgery, David Geffen School of Medicine at UCLA, 10833 Le Conte Avenue, Los Angeles, CA 90095, USA; [c] Division of Surgical Oncology, Department of Surgery, David Geffen School of Medicine at UCLA, 10833 Le Conte Avenue, Los Angeles, CA 90095, USA
* Corresponding author.
E-mail address: Jeffrey.Farma@fccc.edu

the surgical management of melanoma, which has been guided by astute clinical observations and rigorous clinical trials. More conservative margins are now considered adequate and routine complete lymph node dissections have been abandoned since the adoption of sentinel node (SN) biopsy. SN biopsy improves assessment of prognosis and in about 80% to 85% cases it also obviates complete lymph node dissections.[2]

The goal of surgical treatment continues to be eradication of the primary lesion to achieve negative margins and assessment and treatment of regional spread to minimize the chances of local and locoregional relapse. This article details the rationale for margins of excision and discusses the surgical management of locally recurrent melanoma.

DIAGNOSTIC BIOPSY TECHNIQUES

Diagnostic biopsy of a pigmented lesion can be performed in multiple ways (**Table 1**). Excisional biopsy is the preferred method of evaluation of a pigmented lesion. Preliminary excision with 1- to 3-mm margins is considered desirable for appropriate diagnosis and treatment planning. Not only does it give direction regarding final excision margins, but measurement of depth, presence of ulceration, or high mitotic rate can also give direction regarding possibility of metastases to lymph nodes. This may warrant lymphatic mapping and SN biopsy.

However, in practice, other techniques of biopsy, such as incisional biopsy, shave biopsy, or punch biopsy, are commonly used. Biopsy technique has been debated because of the accuracy of these alternative methods of biopsy. The point of debate focuses not only on the completeness of diagnosis from these biopsies, but also the possibility that disruption of tumor may portend worse oncologic outcomes.

One of the earlier studies looked at 193 patients recorded in the California Tumor Registry treated between 1950 and 1954. Initial biopsies were performed in 115 patients and 55 were radically excised. The 10-year overall survival was 65.4% in the biopsy group versus 55.8% for those with initial complete excision. However, the study was limited in that only diameter of the lesion was recorded. Tumor thickness as a prognostic variable was not yet understood, and therefore not recorded.[5]

Table 1 Biopsy techniques		
Type of Biopsy	**Description**	**Utility**
Excisional biopsy	Remove the lesion with 1- to 3-mm margins. Can be performed as an elliptical biopsy, a punch, or saucerization.	Preferred method of biopsy for pigmented lesions.
Incisional biopsy	A full-thickness biopsy of the thickest portion of the lesion.	Useful in certain anatomic areas, such as the face, ear, palm, sole, or digit; and in very large lesions.
Punch biopsy	A full-thickness biopsy that could be excisional if the lesion is very small.	Like incisional biopsy, it is useful if the lesion is large, or if the location is on the face or hand.
Shave biopsy	Involves removal of the superficial layers of the skin with a sharp blade.	Not the preferred method of biopsy. Performed in areas where the index of suspicion is low. Risk of incomplete depth analysis.

Rampen and colleagues[6] looked at incisional biopsies and reported that the risk of local tumor recurrence and metastatic potential may be increased by incisional procedures, by pushing tumor cells to the deep dermis or subcutaneous structures. In this small series of 76 patients, 14 patients who had incisional biopsies had reduced survival compared with 62 patients who had excisional biopsies. However, the authors did not stratify for other predictive factors. Austin and colleagues[7] reported 48 cases of incisional biopsy for head and neck melanoma and reported a significant reduction of survival when compared with the excisional biopsy group. The median follow-up for this study was 36 months, and the only significant difference in either group was that patients in the incisional biopsy group were significantly older. They did not find any difference in local or regional recurrence. In contrast, a study by Griffiths and Briggs[8] retrospectively analyzed 281 patients with clinical stage I invasive cutaneous melanoma from a period of 1967 to 1972 at the Frenchay Hospital in Bristol. They did not find any significant difference in outcome between patients who had received an incisional biopsy, minimal margin excisional biopsy, or primary wide excisional surgery.

Twenty years later, a study by Martin and colleagues[9] looked at a subgroup of 215 patients with head and neck melanomas, and failed to show any significant differences in positive nodes, disease-free, distant disease-free, or overall survival among the excisional, incisional, or shave biopsy groups. Lederman and Sober[10] looked prospectively at 472 patients with clinical stage I cutaneous melanoma, 353 had undergone total excisional biopsies and 119 had punch biopsies or partial excisions. All patients were grouped by four tumor thickness categories. Within these categories there was no significant difference between the incisional and the excisional biopsy groups. The authors recommended incisional biopsies for large lesions or for lesions located in cosmetically sensitive areas. Lees and Briggs[11] performed a large retrospective study in 1991 that included 1086 patients. Of these 990 received a complete excision and 96 had an incisional biopsy. They stratified patients for age, gender, and tumor thickness and found no difference in mortality rates during a 5-year period.

Bong and colleagues[12] evaluated 265 patients who had incisional biopsies, and matched to 469 cases of excisional biopsies from the database of the Scottish Melanoma Group. They found no difference in recurrence or disease-free survival. Molenkamp and colleagues[13] looked at 471 patients who were stage I/II melanoma and underwent re-excision and a SN biopsy. They found that age, Breslow thickness, lymphatic invasion, and SN status were the most consistent and independent confounders of disease-free survival and overall survival. The site of primary melanoma and ulceration were also important confounders of survival. However, both the diagnostic biopsy type and presence of residual tumor cells in the re-excision specimen did not have a negative influence on disease-free and overall survival. With the rising incidence of melanoma, it is important for clinicians to be able to obtain a biopsy diagnosis, although incisional biopsy is not recommended; the presence of positive margins on excisional biopsy need not be considered a failure.

The underlying theme in all of the previously mentioned studies was that although an incisional biopsy or punch biopsy has not been shown to cause a worse disease-free and overall survival, it certainly carries the potential for a considerable sampling error and inaccurate histopathologic diagnosis leading to inaccurate staging. Also, although a shave biopsy has generally been condemned in the diagnosis of melanoma, a deep saucerization performed by an experienced clinician can be adequate.[9] As a surgeon, it is key to adequately review the pathologic information, because in some instances a shave biopsy is adequate, but in others a repeat biopsy may be warranted, if it would change surgical treatment planning and management. The type of biopsy performed depends on the preference of the clinician, and size and location of the lesion.

DEFINITIVE SURGICAL MANAGEMENT: EXCISION MARGINS

Preventing local recurrence and maximizing disease-free and overall survival is the primary aim of surgery. The secondary aims include preserving function and cosmesis with minimal surgical morbidity and minimal hospital stay. Hence the debate has always been about what constitutes an adequate margin width. Early teachings come from Joseph Coats and Herbert Snow in the 1880s and William Handley in the early 1900s. They advocated extensive excision of the primary tumor and a fairly radical regional lymph node dissection. This viewpoint was reinforced by Olsen's[14] report in 1967 in approximately 500 patients, suggesting that atypical melanocytes were often found within 5 cm of the primary melanoma. She emphasized resection with wide margins to encompass these atypical melanocytes. Local recurrence was considered more likely with narrow excision.

The understanding of local recurrence has evolved and a variety of mechanisms explain the pathogenesis of local recurrence. Incomplete excision of the original tumor or persistent disease occurs rarely with wide local excision, but is seen occasionally when anatomic constraints require narrow margin excision or when Mohs surgery is used. An alternate mechanism relates to dissemination of tumor through the intradermal lymphatics. The latter is the more common form and portends a worse overall survival. This indicates systemic involvement, and the unlikely chance that wider excision would be curative.[15] With the understanding that depth of tumor is a bad prognostic indicator compared with the diameter, the dogma of radical wide excision was challenged.

Several large retrospective studies in the 1980s indicated that the risk for local recurrence was low if the tumor was excised with 2-cm margins or more. These studies demonstrated that Breslow thickness was the most important pathologic variable to predict prognosis (**Table 2**). One study came from the Sydney Melanoma Unit in 1985.[21] It determined the recurrence rates in 1839 patients who underwent long-term follow-up. For thick tumors, greater than or equal to 3 mm, the local recurrence rate was 21% when the excision margin was less than 2 cm and 9% when the excision

Table 2
Randomized trials for excision margins

Trial	Author, Year	N	Tumor Thickness (mm)	Excision Margins Compared	Actuarial 5 y Survival
British Association of Plastic Surgeons, UK Melanoma Study Group	Thomas et al,[16] 2004	900	≥2.0	1 vs 3 cm	NR
French Group of Research on Malignant Melanoma Trial	Khayat et al,[17] 2003	337	≤2.0	2 vs 5 cm	93%
Intergroup Melanoma Trial	Balch et al,[18] 1993	468	1.0–4.0	2 vs 4 cm	76
Swedish Melanoma Study Group Trial	Cohn- Cedermark et al,[19] 2000	989	0.8–2.0	2 vs 5 cm	86
World Health Organization melanoma trial	Veronesi &Cascinelli,[20] 1991	612	≤2.0	1 vs 3 cm	97

Data from Refs.[16–20]

margin was 2 cm or more. For thin tumors, 0.1 to 0.7 mm, the local recurrence rates were 2% when excision margins were less than 2 cm and less than 1% when excision margins of 2 cm or more were used.

RANDOMIZED TRIALS FOR MARGINS OF EXCISION

Eventually, large prospective randomized trials were undertaken to clarify the excision margins required to minimize local recurrences and achieve optimal survival outcomes. The World Health Organization Melanoma Program performed a trial in 612 patients with primary melanomas less than 2 mm in thickness, and who had excision of the tumors with either 1- or 3-cm margins.[20] There was no difference in disease-free and overall survival in the two groups; however, local recurrences were higher (3.3%) in melanomas between 1.1 and 2 mm thickness that underwent a narrow excision. Thus, it was concluded that melanomas less than or equal to 1 mm could be adequately treated with a margin of 1 cm. For tumors between 1 and 2 mm thickness, some evidence suggests that excision margins of more than 1 cm are desirable, but this evidence is not conclusive.[22]

The Intergroup Melanoma Surgical Trial in the United States randomized patients with intermediate thickness melanomas (1–4 mm) to be treated with either 2- or 4-cm margins.[18] The recurrence rates were similar for both groups and no significant difference in 5-year survival was seen. The group with 4-cm margins did have significantly greater morbidity and length of hospital stay. Local recurrence was found to be six- to eight-fold higher in patients with ulcerated melanomas.

Similar trials were undertaken in Europe. The Swedish Study Group looked at 989 patients who had melanoma between 0.8 and 2.0 mm in thickness.[19] The French Group for Research on Malignant Melanoma analyzed 326 patients with melanomas 2 mm or more in Breslow thickness.[17] Both studies did not show any evidence that 5-cm margins reduced the local recurrence rate or improved outcome. Another large trial was undertaken in Britain: 900 patients who had melanomas 2 mm or more underwent wide excision with margins of 1 versus 3 cm.[16] They reported that a 1-cm margin was associated with a slightly increased risk of locoregional recurrence compared with a 3-cm margin, but after a median follow-up period of 16 months, no difference in survival outcome was seen.

A systematic review of the previously mentioned randomized trials has been done.[22–24] There are limitations to the meta-analysis given the heterogeneity of these papers. There seems to be clear direction for thin melanomas (<1 mm), with recommendation of 1-cm margins of excision. However, the data are not as definitive for intermediate thickness (1–4 mm) and thick (>4 mm) melanomas. Current guidelines in countries across the world (United States, United Kingdom, Australia, Switzerland, The Netherlands, and Germany) accept a margin of 0.5 to 1 cm for melanoma in situ, 1 cm for thin, and 2 cm for intermediate and thick melanomas (**Table 3**). Further

Table 3
Recommended margin of excision

Breslow Thickness (mm)	T Stage	Recommended Margin of Excision (cm)
Melanoma in situ	Tis	0.5–1
<1.0	T1	1
1.01–2.0	T2	1–2
2.01–4.0	T3	2
>4.0	T4	2

trials have been deemed necessary to define the role of narrower margins of excision, and their impact on local recurrence and overall survival.[25]

Recently, Pasquali and colleagues[26] analyzed a group of 632 patients with clinically lymph node–negative melanomas, more than 4 mm thick. A total of 397 patients had a SN biopsy in addition to wide excision to at least a 2-cm clinical margin (corresponding to a 16-mm histopathologic margin). Of note, patients who did not undergo SN biopsy were enrolled in the observation arm of the Multicenter Selective Lymphadenectomy Trial-1. Their study concluded that histopathologically determined primary tumor margins more than 16 mm, corresponding to surgical 2-cm margins, were associated with better local control in melanomas greater than 4 mm thick. Patients achieved the best local and locoregional control when SN biopsy was coupled with the greater than 16-mm histologic excision margin. This study highlights that improvement in local and locoregional control may be a reflection not only of wide margins, but also of inclusion of SN biopsy.

LOCAL RECURRENCE OF MELANOMA

Local recurrence of melanoma has been ambiguously described in the literature and thus encompasses a spectrum of disease processes occurring within the vicinity of the primary tumor.[27] Brown and Zitelli[28] described a series of patients with "true local cutaneous recurrent malignant melanoma," defined as melanoma arising contiguous with the scar from the primary excision, likely resulting from inadequate excision of the primary tumor; the prognosis in this series was generally excellent and related to the thickness of the primary tumor. In contrast, Roses and colleagues[29] reported that 90% of patients with "local metastasis," defined as biopsy-proved metastatic disease within a distance of 5 cm from the perimeter of the primary scar or skin graft, ultimately developed systemic metastases. The current and most widely accepted definition of local recurrence of melanoma is regrowth within 2 cm of the surgical scar after a definitive excision of the primary melanoma with appropriate surgical margins.[18] Although this is a somewhat arbitrary definition, it has been consistently used as an end point in most recent prospective randomized trials. Local recurrence frequently indicatives aggressive tumor biology and is associated with significant morbidity and mortality.

Risk Factors, Epidemiology, and Survival

The overall rate of local recurrence in contemporary studies approaches 4%.[16,30] The risk factors for local recurrence have been well-documented in the Intergroup Melanoma Trial. Increasing tumor thickness and tumor ulceration are the primary risk factors for local recurrence.[30,31] Local recurrences are seen more frequently with melanomas of the distal extremity (5.2%) and head and neck (9.4%) compared with melanomas of the proximal extremities (1.7%) or trunk (2.7%).[30] Most local recurrences (70%) occurred within 5 years of follow-up and patients with thicker lesions or ulcerated melanomas tended to develop local recurrences earlier.[30] Previous concerns that the SN biopsy procedure may predispose patients to developing local recurrence of melanoma have been allayed by the MSLT-1 trial, which demonstrated no difference in local recurrence rates for patients undergoing SN biopsy versus observation. In addition, MSLT-1 demonstrated that patients with a positive SN were at higher risk for local or in-transit recurrences.[32,33]

Surgical margins wider than 2 cm clearly do not decrease the risk of local recurrence; however, it remains unclear whether a 1-cm margin provides adequate local control. The Intergroup Melanoma Trial demonstrated equivalent local recurrence rates in the comparison of 2- with 4-cm surgical margins.[30,31] In the World Health

Organization trial comparing 1- with 3-cm surgical margins in patients with melanoma less than or equal to 2 cm in thickness, local recurrences were seen in 3 of 305 patients randomized to undergo excision with 1-cm margins and no local recurrences were documented in the 310 patients randomized to the 3-cm margin arm. All of the local recurrences occurred in patients with melanomas at least 1 cm thickness.[30] In the United Kingdom Melanoma Study Group trial, 900 patients with melanomas at least 2 mm in thickness were randomized to excision with 1- versus 3-cm surgical margins. Locoregional recurrences (nodal, in transit, and local recurrences) were more frequent in the group randomized to a 1-cm margin (168 of 453 patients) compared with the 3-cm margin cohort (142 of 447 patients). This difference was statistically significant, but it should be noted that the rates of isolated local recurrence (excluding nodal recurrences) between the 1- and 3-cm study groups were not statistically different (3.9% vs 3.4%).[16]

Local recurrence portends a poor prognosis. The 5- and 10-year survival for patients with local recurrence in the Intergroup Melanoma Trial was 9% and 5%, respectively.[31] These patients had high rates of subsequent development of in-transit metastasis, nodal metastasis, and distant hematogenous dissemination.[30,31] The survival data clearly demonstrate that most local recurrences exhibit aggressive biologic behavior that is akin to metastatic melanoma.

Management

Patients presenting with local recurrence are evaluated with a detailed history and physical examination. A biopsy should be obtained to confirm recurrence. Because regional and distant metastases are common, thorough imaging is justified. The most common imaging modalities used are computed tomography of the head, chest, abdomen, pelvis, and the site of recurrence versus whole body positron emission tomography and consideration for brain MRI. Special attention should be paid to the soft tissues in the vicinity of the recurrence where in-transit metastases may be difficult to detect clinically and radiographically.

For patients who are adherent to scheduled follow-up, local recurrences are frequently detected at a size amenable to surgical resection. Despite the high probability of regional and distant metastases, treatment of the site of recurrence is indicated for local control and to obtain tissue for pathologic analysis including mutation status. There is great variability in survival outcomes among the different published reports, but it is clear that a subset of patients do enjoy long disease-free survival after resection of local recurrences and some are likely cured of the disease. Thus, surgical resection should be considered when feasible. There are limited data to define the principles of resection, but most experts recommend approximately 1-cm margins with the goal of obtaining microscopically negative margins. Primary closure is preferable, but skin grafting or other methods of complex closure are frequently required at surgical sites where adequate wide local excision has previously been performed.

Yao and colleagues[34] have reported their experience with lymphatic mapping and SN biopsy in the setting of recurrent melanoma. In this series of 30 patients with in-transit and recurrent melanoma, SNs could be accurately identified in every patient including the 10 patients who had prior lymph node surgery. Approximately half of the patients had positive SNs and some subsequently underwent regional lymphadenectomy. This study demonstrates that a SN biopsy is feasible in this patient population. No statistically significant differences were detected in overall survival between the node-negative and node-positive patients. This approach provides more thorough staging, but it remains unclear whether the procedure has therapeutic value in the setting of recurrent melanoma.

For some patients with local recurrence, resection may not be feasible because of the extent of disease, anatomic location, or patient-related factors. Alternative efforts to treat the local recurrence are still important because these disease sites often progress and can be a source of significant morbidity and may negatively impact quality of life. These patients may be considered for intratumoral therapies, isolated limb perfusion or infusion, radiation therapy, systemic therapies, or clinical trials.

In summary, the mainstay of treatment of melanoma is surgery. Lifelong surveillance is crucial because of the risk of (1) second primary melanomas, (2) locoregional recurrence, (3) late recurrence, and (4) other cutaneous malignancies. Risk of local recurrence is greatest in the first 5 years after diagnosis, especially in thick and ulcerated tumors. Current recommendations, based on randomized trials, dictate appropriate margin width based on the depth of the primary melanoma.

REFERENCES

1. DeSantis CE, Lin CC, Mariotto AB, et al. Cancer treatment and survivorship statistics, 2014. CA Cancer J Clin 2014;64(4):252–71.
2. Thompson JF, Scolyer RA, Uren RF. Surgical management of primary cutaneous melanoma: excision margins and the role of sentinel lymph node examination. Surg Oncol Clin N Am 2006;15(2):301–18.
3. Pringle JH. A method of operation in melanotic tumours of the skin. Edinb Med J 1908;23:496–9.
4. Hogarth Pringle J. Cutaneous melanoma two cases alive thirty and thirty-eight years after operation. Lancet 1937;229(5922):508–9.
5. Epstein E, Bragg K, Linden G. Biopsy and prognosis of malignant melanoma. JAMA 1969;208(8):1369–71.
6. Rampen FH, van Houten WA, Jop WC. Incisional procedures and prognosis in malignant melanoma. Clin Exp Dermatol 1980;5(3):313–20.
7. Austin JR, Byers RM, Brown WD, et al. Influence of biopsy on the prognosis of cutaneous melanoma of the head and neck. Head Neck 1996;18(2):107–17.
8. Griffiths RW, Briggs JC. Biopsy procedures, primary wide excisional surgery and long term prognosis in primary clinical stage I invasive cutaneous malignant melanoma. Ann R Coll Surg Engl 1985;67(2):75–8.
9. Martin RC II, Scoggins CR, Ross MI, et al. Is incisional biopsy of melanoma harmful? Am J Surg 2005;190(6):913–7.
10. Lederman JS, Sober AJ. Does biopsy type influence survival in clinical stage I cutaneous melanoma? J Am Acad Dermatol 1985;13(6):983–7.
11. Lees VC, Briggs JC. Effect of initial biopsy procedure on prognosis in stage 1 invasive cutaneous malignant melanoma: review of 1086 patients. Br J Surg 1991;78(9):1108–10.
12. Bong JL, Herd RM, Hunter JA. Incisional biopsy and melanoma prognosis. J Am Acad Dermatol 2002;46(5):690–4.
13. Molenkamp BG, Sluijter BJ, Oosterhof B, et al. Non-radical diagnostic biopsies do not negatively influence melanoma patient survival. Ann Surg Oncol 2007;14(4):1424–30.
14. Olsen G. The malignant melanoma of the skin. New theories based on a study of 500 cases. Dan Med Bull 1967;14(9):229–38.
15. Heenan PJ. Local recurrence of melanoma. Pathology 2004;36(5):491–5.
16. Thomas JM, Newton-Bishop J, A'Hern R, et al. Excision margins in high-risk malignant melanoma. N Engl J Med 2004;350(8):757–66.

17. Khayat D, Rixe O, Martin G, et al. Surgical margins in cutaneous melanoma (2 cm versus 5 cm for lesions measuring less than 2.1-mm thick). Cancer 2003;97(8): 1941–6.
18. Balch CM, Urist MM, Karakousis CP, et al. Efficacy of 2-cm surgical margins for intermediate-thickness melanomas (1 to 4 mm). Results of a multi-institutional randomized surgical trial. Ann Surg 1993;218(3):262–7 [discussion: 267–9].
19. Balch CM, Urist MM, Karakousis CP, et al. Long term results of a randomized study by the Swedish Melanoma Study Group on 2-cm versus 5-cm resection margins for patients with cutaneous melanoma with a tumor thickness of 0.8–2.0 mm. Cancer 2000;89(7):1495–501.
20. Veronesi U, Cascinelli N. Narrow excision (1-cm margin). A safe procedure for thin cutaneous melanoma. Arch Surg 1991;126(4):438–41.
21. Milton GW, Shaw HM, McCarthy WH. Resection margins for melanoma. Aust N Z J Surg 1985;55(3):225–6.
22. Haigh PI, DiFronzo LA, McCready DR. Optimal excision margins for primary cutaneous melanoma: a systematic review and meta-analysis. Can J Surg 2003;46(6): 419–26.
23. Sladden MJ, Balch C, Barzilai DA, et al. Surgical excision margins for primary cutaneous melanoma. Cochrane Database Syst Rev 2009;(4):CD004835.
24. Lens MB, Dawes M, Goodacre T, et al. Excision margins in the treatment of primary cutaneous melanoma: a systematic review of randomized controlled trials comparing narrow vs wide excision. Arch Surg 2002;137(10):1101–5.
25. Johnson TM, Sondak VK. Melanoma margins: the importance and need for more evidence-based trials. Arch Dermatol 2004;140(9):1148–50.
26. Pasquali S, Haydu LE, Scolyer RA, et al. The importance of adequate primary tumor excision margins and sentinel node biopsy in achieving optimal locoregional control for patients with thick primary melanomas. Ann Surg 2013;258(1):152–7.
27. MacCormack MA, Cohen LM, Rogers GS. Local melanoma recurrence: a clarification of terminology. Dermatol Surg 2004;30(12 Pt 2):1533–8.
28. Brown CD, Zitelli JA. The prognosis and treatment of true local cutaneous recurrent malignant melanoma. Dermatol Surg 1995;21(4):285–90.
29. Roses DF, Harris MN, Riquel D, et al. Local and in-transit metastases following definitive excision for primary cutaneous malignant melanoma. Ann Surg 1983; 198(1):65–9.
30. Karakousis CP, Balch CM, Urist MM, et al. Local recurrence in malignant melanoma: long-term results of the multiinstitutional randomized surgical trial. Ann Surg Oncol 1996;3(5):446–52.
31. Balch CM, Soong SJ, Ross MI, et al. Long-term results of a prospective surgical trial comparing 2 cm vs. 4 cm excision margins for 740 patients with 1-4 mm melanomas. Ann Surg Oncol 2001;8(2):101–8.
32. Morton DL, Thompson JF, Cochran AJ, et al. Sentinel-node biopsy or nodal observation in melanoma. N Engl J Med 2006;355(13):1307–17.
33. Morton DL, Thompson JF, Cochran AJ, et al. Final trial report of sentinel-node biopsy versus nodal observation in melanoma. N Engl J Med 2014;370(7):599–609.
34. Yao KA, Hsueh EC, Essner R, et al. Is sentinel lymph node mapping indicated for isolated local and in-transit recurrent melanoma? Ann Surg 2003;238(5):743–7.

Sentinel Lymph Node Mapping in Melanoma in the Twenty-first Century

Matthew P. Doepker, MD, Jonathan S. Zager, MD*

KEYWORDS

- Sentinel lymph node biopsy • Lymphoscintigraphy • Melanoma • Thin • Thick
- Desmoplastic

KEY POINTS

- More than 76,000 cases of melanoma were diagnosed in 2013, with most of those cases being thin melanoma (≤1.0 mm).
- The standard of care in staging the regional nodal basin in patients with intermediate-thickness melanoma (1.01–4.0 mm) is sentinel lymph node biopsy.
- Thin melanomas (0.76–1.0 mm) as well as thick melanomas (>4.0 mm) should be considered for a sentinel lymph node biopsy.
- The addition of newer radiocolloids and single-photon emission computed tomography lymphoscintigraphy may help improve the accuracy of finding sentinel lymph nodes.

The incidence of melanoma is increasing faster than any other cancer, with an estimated lifetime risk of 1 in 53. In the United States in 2013, more than 76,690 cases of invasive melanoma were diagnosed with an estimated 9480 deaths from the disease.[1] The most common site of melanoma metastasis involves the regional nodal basin and the status of the sentinel lymph node (SLN) has been for decades, and still remains, the most important prognostic factor in the diagnosis of melanoma.[2] SLN biopsy (SLNB) has been to shown to be highly accurate with low morbidity and is currently recommended to be performed for staging in patients diagnosed with an intermediate-thickness melanoma (1.01–4.0 mm), as summarized in **Table 1**.[2–4] SLNB has been the subject of controversy, especially when used to stage thin (≤1 mm), thick (>4 mm), or desmoplastic melanomas (DM). This article reviews the current literature regarding the use of SLNB in thin, intermediate, and thick melanoma, and in DM. Data supporting the use of newer radiopharmaceuticals and colorimetric

Disclosure: The authors have nothing to disclose.
Department of Cutaneous Oncology, Moffitt Cancer Center, 12902 Magnolia Drive SRB-4, Tampa, FL 33612, USA
* Corresponding author.
E-mail address: jonathan.zager@moffitt.org

Table 1
SLNB recommendations based on National Comprehensive Cancer Network (NCCN) guidelines

Melanoma Thickness (mm)	NCCN Recommendations Regarding SLNB
Melanoma in situ	Not recommended
<0.76	Not recommended
0.76–1.0 (no ulceration and mitotic rate <1/mm^2)	Considered
0.76–1.0 (ulcerated or mitotic rate ≥1/mm^2)	Discussed and offered
≥1.0–4.0	Discussed and offered

agents in SLN mapping, along with newer imaging modalities to identify SLNs, are also reviewed.

RANDOMIZED TRIALS OF SENTINEL LYMPH NODE BIOPSY IN MELANOMA

The role of SLNB in melanoma has been evaluated by several large, prospective, randomized trials. The Multicenter Selective Lymphadenectomy Trial (MSLT-I) was a prospective, randomized trial designed with the goal of determining whether SLNB provided a survival benefit to patients with primary melanoma. The Sunbelt Melanoma Trial, another prospective, randomized trial, was also designed to evaluate survival after SLNB, as well as the benefit of adjuvant interferon (IFN) alfa-2b toward overall survival (OS) or disease-free survival (DFS). The Multicenter Selective Lymphadenectomy Trial II (MSLT-II), which has reached its accrual goal in 2014 and is currently in the follow-up stage, was designed to determine whether a completion lymph node dissection (CLND) of the affected nodal basin was necessary after detection of a positive SLNB, with the intent to determine whether CLND has any benefit in regional control or OS.[5,6]

   MSLT-I began patient accrual in 1994 and reached its target of 2001 patients in March of 2002. The final analysis was published in early 2014. The patients were randomly assigned to either undergo wide local excision (WLE) alone with observation of the nodal basin or WLE with SLNB and immediate CLND if there was a positive SLN. The trial evaluated 1347 patients with intermediate-thickness melanomas (1.2–3.5 mm). Final analysis showed no difference between the SLN and observation groups with respect to melanoma-specific survival (MSS) at 10 years (81.4% and 78.3%; hazard ratio [HR], 0.84; P = .18). Improvement in 10-year DFS of 71.3% versus 64.7% (HR, 0.76; P = .01) in favor of the SLN group was reported. Patients who had SLN metastasis had worse outcomes than those who were SLN negative, with a 10-year MSS of 62.1% versus 85.1% for SLN positive versus negative, respectively (HR, 3.09; P<.001). On multivariate analysis, the investigators reported that SLN status was the strongest predictor of recurrence or death from melanoma. Patients with SLN metastasis who received immediate CLND were compared with those in the observation group who failed in the nodal basin with clinically obvious disease, with distant DFS being significantly improved in favor of the SLN-positive group (54.8% vs 35.6%; HR, 0.62; P = .02). Of those with nodal metastasis, the 10-year MSS was significantly improved in favor of the those with a positive SLN versus those who failed clinically in the nodal basin in the observation group (62.1% vs 41.5%; HR, 0.56; P = .006). The MSLT-I trial concluded that the use of SLNB in intermediate-thickness melanoma is not only feasible; it improves DFS and decreases the risk of nodal recurrence and distant metastasis. MSS was significantly improved in those with SLN metastasis compared with those observed with clinical nodal failure, supporting that detection of nodal metastases at an occult stage via SLNB is beneficial.[7–10]

The Sunbelt Melanoma Trial is a multicenter prospective randomized trial to evaluate the role of high-dose IFN-α2b or observation (no adjuvant therapy) in patients who had a CLND after a positive SLNB. The trial also evaluated the impact of reverse transcription polymerase chain reaction (RT-PCR)–positive SLNs that were initially negative by standard histology and immunohistochemistry (IHC), and then found to be positive on RT-PCR for tyrosinase and at least 1 other marker (MART-1, gp 100, or MAGE-3). Those patients who were SLNB positive by RT-PCR were randomized to observation, CLND, or CLND plus IFN-α.[11] The final analysis included 774 patients with a median follow-up of 64 months. The patients who were randomized to IFN groups received treatments for a total of 52 weeks. Primary end points of the study were OS and DFS. No statistical significant difference was seen in OS (HR, 1.07; $P = .79$) or DFS (HR, 0.82; $P = .46$) in patients randomized to either IFN or observation. No statistical significant benefit was reported among those found to be positive by RT-PCR analysis treated with CLND, CLND plus IFN-α, or observation. This study concluded that there was no additional benefit for the addition of IFN-α after undergoing a CLND for SLN-positive disease detected by hematoxylin and eosin or IHC, and in those patients in whom SLN disease was detected by RT-PCR there was no benefit to CLND or CLND plus IFN.[11,12]

Although the current standard of care is to perform a CLND for patients with a positive SLN, only about 15% to 18% of completion lymphadenectomy specimens after SLNB contain additional nodes with metastatic disease (ie, nonsentinel nodes).[7,13–17] MSLT-II was designed to determine whether CLND is necessary in patients with a positive SLN. The primary outcome of MSLT-II is MSS. The secondary outcomes are OS; DFS; prognostic accuracy of histopathology; molecular and immunologic markers; and quality of life.[5] The study commenced in December 2004 and has just reached its accrual goal of 1925 patients (in early 2014). Patients with a positive SLNB are randomly assigned either to undergo immediate CLND or observation with high-resolution ultrasonography every 4 months for 2 years; every 6 months for years 3, 4, and 5; and yearly thereafter.[2,6]

COMPLICATIONS ASSOCIATED WITH SENTINEL LYMPH NODE BIOPSY

The use of SLNB has supplanted the use of elective CLND and become the standard of care around the world in patients with primary, localized melanomas. CLND can be associated with increased morbidity with the most common complications being wound infection, seroma/hematoma, lymphedema, pain, and numbness.[18,19] The incidence of these complications is significantly higher in CLND compared with SLNB. This difference has been addressed in several trials, including MSLT-I and The Sunbelt Melanoma Trial. In MSLT-I, complications occurred in 10.1% of patients undergoing just SLNB, compared with 37.2% with the addition of CLND.[18] The Sunbelt Melanoma Trial also compared SLNB and SLNB plus CLND and showed higher rates of wound infection (1.1% vs 7.0%), lymphedema (0.7% vs 11.7%), and seroma/hematoma (2.3% vs 5.9%) with SLNB plus CLND.[9,10,19,20] There have been reports of allergic reactions after the use blue dye, especially isosulfan blue dye. MSLT-I reported only a 0.2% incidence of allergic reaction to isosulfan blue dye when used for SLNB. In general, SLNB is a safe procedure that yields accurate results for patients diagnosed with early-stage melanoma.

MANAGEMENT OF THIN MELANOMA

No consensus in the literature exists on whether to perform SLNB in patients with thin melanoma (≤ 1 mm). The American Society of Clinical Oncology and Society of Surgical Oncology (ASCO/SSO), along with the National Comprehensive Cancer Network (NCCN), recommend consideration of SLNB in certain patients with thin melanomas, not routine use as recommended in patients with intermediate-thickness melanomas (see **Table 1**).[3,4,21,22] Some clinicians argue against SLNB in thin melanoma because of the reported low rate of nodal metastases (<5%),[23,24] whereas others report a higher than 5% incidence of nodal metastasis in thin melanomas.[25–29]

Kesmodel and colleagues[29] conducted a retrospective single-institution review of 181 patients with thin melanomas (≤1 mm) over an 8-year period. Univariate and multivariate logistic regression analysis was performed to identify clinical and histopathologic variables in thin melanoma associated with an increased risk for SLN positivity. Age, sex, anatomic location, mitotic rate (MR), thickness, Clark level, and ulceration were examined. MR and Clark level were further defined as 0 or more than 0 mitoses and level II/III or IV/V, respectively. The overall reported SLN positivity rate was 5% for the sample cohort analyzed. Both MR ($P =.011$) and tumor thickness (≥0.76 mm) ($P = .033$) were significant for SLN positivity on univariate analysis. On multiple regression analysis, only MR remained significant. The investigators concluded that MR was a predictor of SLN metastasis in thin melanoma and could be used to help determine which patients with thin melanomas (≤1 mm) should undergo SLNB and are at higher risk for SLN metastases.

More recently, Han and colleagues[28] assessed 271 patients with thin melanomas to determine factors predictive of nodal metastasis. Clinicopathologic factors that were evaluated included age, Breslow thickness, Clark level, regression, ulceration, MR, positive deep biopsy sample margin, vertical growth phase (VGP), tumor-infiltrating lymphocytes (TILs), and the American Joint Committee on Cancer (AJCC) T classification. The overall median Breslow thickness was 0.85 mm (range, 0.3–1.0 mm; P = nonsignificant). Of the 271 patients, 22 (8.1%) had a positive SLN. Melanomas were also classified as either T1a or T1b. Five percent of T1a melanomas (no ulceration, and $MR<1/mm^2$) had positive SLNs, whereas 13% of patients with T1b melanomas (ulcerated and/or MR $\geq1/mm^2$) had a positive SLN. Multiple logistic regression analysis showed that ulceration significantly correlated with SLN metastasis ($P<.05$) and MR greater than or equal to $1/mm^2$ significantly correlated with any nodal metastasis ($P<.05$) including recurrent regional nodal disease. Age, Clark level, regression, positive deep biopsy sample margin, TIL, and VGP were not significant predictors of either clinically positive nodal disease or SLN metastasis. SLN metastasis was seen in 8.4% of all thin melanomas greater than or equal to 0.76 mm, whereas 6.1% of those less than 0.76 mm had a positive SLN (both SLN-positive patients in the <0.76 mm group had T1b melanomas). From these results the investigators concluded that it is justifiable to consider and perform SLNB in patients with tumors greater than or equal to 0.76 mm. The investigators concluded that, in the absence of ulceration, there is no clear indication for SLNB in melanomas less than 0.76 mm.

The same group followed up with a larger retrospective review of a multi-institutional database of 1250 patients with thin melanoma (≤1 mm) from 1994 to 2012 to determine which clinicopathologic factors increase the risk of SLN metastasis in patients with thin melanomas.[23] Clinicopathologic factors analyzed in this study were Breslow thickness, Clark level, ulceration, MR, regression, VGP, lymphovascular invasion, and TILs. Median follow-up was 2.6 years. On univariate analysis, Breslow thickness, Clark level, ulceration, and MR were significantly different between SLN-positive and SLN-negative groups. On multiple logistic regression analysis, Breslow thickness greater than or equal to 0.75 mm (P = .03), Clark level greater than or equal to IV (P = .05), and ulceration (P = .01) predicted SLN metastasis. The overall risk was 5.2%, but it increased to 6.3% in tumors greater than or equal to 0.75 mm. Although varying values of MR have been reported in several studies to be predictive of SLN metastasis, an MR of greater than or equal to $1.0/mm^2$ did not predict SLN metastasis in melanoma in this study ($P = .98$).[30–32] Of all SLN-positive patients, 86.2% had a thickness greater than or equal to 0.75 mm. Of those patients with a melanoma greater than or equal to 0.75 mm and a positive SLN, more than 90% were ulcerated and/or Clark level greater than or equal to IV. The investigators showed that using only ulceration or Clark level greater than or equal to IV potentially misses 81.7% and 31.6% of SLN-positive patients. They concluded that a 5% risk of metastasis should be used as a threshold for performing SLNB, and this threshold was met in patients with melanomas of greater than or equal to 0.75 mm. Although SLN positivity has been reported in patients with melanomas less than 0.5 mm, none were positive in this study and only 2.5% of those patients with primary melanomas between 0.5 and 0.75 mm had a positive SLN.[33,34]

MANAGEMENT OF THICK MELANOMA

Performing SLNB in patients with thick melanomas, defined as greater than or equal to 4.0 mm, is another area of controversy. Patients with thick melanomas are considered to have a high risk of both regional or distant metastatic disease at presentation (33%–44%).[35] In the past, SLNB was not offered to patients with thick melanoma because of the increased risk of distant metastasis at presentation. Gershenwald and colleagues[36] reviewed 131 patients with primary tumors with a depth of greater than or equal to 4.0 mm who underwent lymphatic mapping and SLNB. Of the 131 patients, 126 had a successful SLNB, with at least 1 SLN being identified. Several prognostic factors were assessed, including tumor thickness, ulceration, Clark level, location, sex, and SLN status. Univariate and multivariate analyses were performed to assess the impact of these factors on OS and DFS. There was a 39% positive SLN rate (49 of 126 patients). The median follow-up was 3 years. Nonulcerated primary tumors and negative SLN status were associated with improved DFS and OS. On multivariate analysis, both ulceration and SLN status remained significant, but SLN status was the strongest predictor of survival. The investigators concluded that performing SLNB in patients with thick melanomas can provide valuable prognostic information and help stratify those who would benefit from adjuvant therapy or participation in a clinical trial.

Cherpelis and colleagues[37] performed a single-institution retrospective review of 201 patients diagnosed with thick melanoma, which was defined as greater than or equal to 3.0 mm. The mean thickness was 5.1 mm. The median follow-up was 51 months, with 180 (90%) patients still alive at follow-up. Fifty-one patients had a positive SLNB (25%). This study evaluated the influence of Breslow thickness, Clark level, MR, and regression and SLN status on DFS and OS. Statistically significant differences in 3-year DFS existed between SLN-positive and SLN-negative groups (37% vs 73%; $P = .02$) and ulcerated and nonulcerated lesions (77% vs 93%; $P = .05$). Three-year OS analysis did not reach statistical significance for either SLN positivity or primary tumor ulceration. The other parameters did not have an influence on OS or DFS. This study showed that SLN-positive disease is an important prognostic indicator in patients with thick melanomas, which can help guide future therapy with CLND, adjuvant treatments, or clinical trials.

The final analysis of MSLT-I evaluated 290 patients with thick melanomas, defined as greater than 3.5 mm in that study. One hundred and seventy-three were randomized to the SLNB group and 117 to the observation group. Fifty-seven (33%) of the 173 in the SLNB group had SLN metastases. Twelve of the 116 SLN negative patients eventually developed nodal disease, bringing the incidence of nodal metastasis in the SLN biopsy group to 39.9%. In the observation group, 44 (37.6%) developed nodal disease at a median of 9.2 months, with the incidence of nodal metastasis increasing to 41.4% at 10-years in the observation group. The 5-year and 10-year cumulative incidences of nodal metastasis were 41% and 42% respectively. The 10-year DFS between the SLN biopsy group and observation group was 50.7% and 40.5% respectively (HR, 0.70; $P = .03$). In patients with thick melanoma and SLN metastasis compared with those without SLN metastases, the 10-year MSS was 48.0% versus 64.6% (HR, 1.75; $P = .03$). However, no statistical significant difference was reported in the distant DFS of patients undergoing immediate versus delayed CLND for nodal metastasis. The final analysis suggests that patients with thick melanoma may benefit from CLND. However, the timing of CLND may not be as critical as in patients with intermediate-thickness melanomas.[7]

MANAGEMENT OF DESMOPLASTIC MELANOMA

The role of SLNB in DM is also controversial. DM is characterized by a proliferation of malignant spindled melanocytes within a collagenous/myxoid stroma, described as desmoplastic.[38] DMs tend to present as thicker tumors, but are often cited in the literature as having lower rates of nodal metastasis.[39–42] DM has been subdivided into the histologic subtypes of pure and mixed variants based on the amount of desmoplasia seen within the tumor. Conflicting reports in the literature cite different rates of nodal metastasis for each subtype.[43–45] NCCN guidelines do not provide any formal recommendations regarding SLNB for DM, whereas the ASCO/SSO guidelines call for SLNB with DM.[3,4] A large, single-institution, retrospective review identified 205 patients with DM who underwent SLNB over an 18-year period. Of the 205 cases, the histologic subtype was known for 128 (67 pure, 61 mixed). The overall median thickness was 3.7 mm (range, 0.5–35 mm), with similar thickness between both subtypes (mixed, 4.4 mm; pure, 4.8 mm). Overall, SLN metastases were seen in 28 patients (13.7%). The SLN positivity rate for mixed and pure variants was 24.6% and 9.0% respectively. Multiple logistic regression analysis showed that histologic subtype correlated with SLN positivity (odds ratio, 3.0 for mixed vs pure; 95% confidence interval, 1.1–8.7; $P<.05$). Patients with a positive SLN also had a significantly higher risk of MSS ($P = .01$). Based on the SLN positivity rate and worse death, the investigators recommended consideration of SLNB for both subtypes.

REPEAT SENTINEL LYMPH NODE BIOPSY AFTER LOCOREGIONAL RECURRENT DISEASE

The value of SLNB has been questioned in patients who develop a locoregional recurrence or in-transit disease. It was originally thought that performing an SLNB would alter and disrupt the lymphatic drainage, rendering a repeat SLNB inaccurate and unreliable.[46–51] A study published in 2003 from Coventry and colleagues[52] included 12 patients who had subcutaneous or cutaneous recurrences after initially having only a WLE. No patient in the study was diagnosed with systemic disease. All recurrences were less than 5 cm from the primary site. All 12 patients had a successful SLNB using both radiocolloid and blue dye for lymphatic mapping. Four (33.3%) patients had a positive SLN. The investigators showed that SLNB is feasible and potentially accurate after WLE. A more recent study by Beasley and colleagues[46] identified 33 patients who initially had a WLE and SLNB for a primary cutaneous melanoma who then either had local or in-transit recurrence. All patients underwent lymphatic mapping, either with technetium 99m sulfur colloid alone (15) or in conjunction with to lymphazurin blue dye (18). Twenty-six patients of the 33 (76%) had a prior SLNB with removal of lymph nodes in the same nodal basin to which the local or in-transit recurrence mapped. At least 1 lymph node was found in 32 of 33 patients (97%). The SLN was positive in 33% of the cases. The investigators showed that SLNB was technically possible and the information gained from this provided prognostic information that could help guide future therapy.

REFINEMENT OF TECHNIQUE AND NEW IMAGING MODALITIES

A gold standard of the agents to use for lymphoscintigraphy (LS) does not exist. The technique of performing SLNB requires the injection of vital blue dyes, either isosulfan blue or patent blue V, alone or in combination with radiocolloid. Surgeons have relied on using radiocolloid preoperatively for LS. It has also been used intraoperatively for identification of nodes using a hand-held gamma probe alone or in combination with blue dye visualized within the afferent lymphatics and the node. Other clinicians prefer to use only radiocolloid, because the supply of vital blue dyes is limited, and one blue dye, methylene blue, has questionable safety and efficacy.[53–56] Few agents have been introduced or have been specifically approved for LS. Recently, a contrast agent, [99mTc]tilmanocept, was designed specifically for the identification of sentinel nodes during intraoperative lymphatic mapping.[57] [99mTc]Tilmanocept is a synthetic macromolecule that binds to the CD206 receptors expressed on reticuloendothelial cells residing in lymph nodes.[58,59] This macromolecule was used and compared with vital blue dye for the localization and identification of SLNs in patients with melanoma.

Two multi-institutional, open-label, prospective, nonrandomized phase III trials compared [99mTc]tilmanocept with vital blue dye in SLN identification. The primary end point in the studies was concordance of [99mTc]tilmanocept with blue dye, with a prespecified minimal concordance level of 90%. Reverse concordance, described as the percentage of radioactive lymph nodes that were also blue, was calculated and reported as a secondary end point. A total of 170 patients with intermediate-thickness melanoma (1.01–4.00 mm) were enrolled in the two phase III trials. The final analysis included 154 patients who were injected with both [99mTc]tilmanocept and blue dye and evaluated intraoperatively. Of the 154 patients who were injected and underwent surgery, 138 had at least 1 blue SLN and 150 had at least 1 radioactive SLN ($P = .002$). Seventy-six of the 150 who were radioactive were also blue. Overall, 379 lymph nodes were excised. Of those, 235 were blue and 364 were radioactive. Of those 235 patients who had a blue node, 232 were radioactive, for a concordance rate of 98.7% ($P<.001$). The reverse concordance was 63.7%, with 364 radioactive nodes being identified, of which 232 were also blue. There were 45 nodes (22.1%) with melanoma detected. [99mTc]Tilmanocept identified all 45 nodes with melanoma compared with only 36 identified (80%) with blue dye alone ($P = .004$).[53] The results of trials show that [99mTc]tilmanocept identified more SLN-containing tumors than blue dye. Adverse events were evaluated, with no reports of immediate or delayed hypersensitivity reactions. Future directions may include setting up trials to compare [99mTc]tilmanocept with other available colloids, or even other imaging modalities, such as single-photon emission computed tomography (SPECT)/computed tomography (CT).

SLNB has been established as a staging procedure and a determinant of prognosis. Using only LS or blue dye can be problematic for surgeons, especially in areas with varied or inconsistent lymphatic drainage areas, such as the back or head and neck region.[60,61] SPECT/CT is an imaging technique that has seen increasing use in the clinical arena. This technique fuses radioactivity distribution detected by SPECT over images produced by the CT scan, which allows surgeons to determine the location of the node in relation to anatomic structures, thus facilitating better operative planning and easier removal. In a prospective trial from the Netherlands, 38 patients diagnosed with head and neck melanomas with a median Breslow thickness of 2.9 mm (range, 0.8–7.8 mm) received conventional LS followed by SPECT/CT. An additional sentinel node was identified in 16% of the patients. All of the anatomic locations of the so-called hot nodes were identified and the surgical approach changed in 11 patients (55%). This study supports the use of SPECT/CT and its advantage of finding the location of the sentinel node, which may help improve the higher false-negative rates of 12% to 44% seen specifically with head and neck melanomas.[18,62–65]

Recently, a retrospective review compared SPECT/CT with planar LS done in the same patients. Ninety-nine consecutive patients (86 had melanoma) underwent both SPECT and planar LS on the day of surgery. Of the 99 patients, 61% had cutaneous malignancies in the head and neck region. The mean numbers of nodes identified on SPECT compared with planar LS were 3.17 and 2.61, respectively ($P<.0001$). Thirty-nine patients (39.4%) had additional nodes seen on SPECT imaging compared with the planar LS. There were 11 patients (11.1%) with additional nodes identified on planar LS not seen on SPECT. Forty-nine (50%) had concordant imaging between both SPECT and planar LS. Because of the risk of missing nodes with either modality, the investigators recommended adding SPECT LS to planar LS to aid in the identification of more draining lymph nodes and potentially to decrease false-negative SLNBs, especially in areas where there might be drainage to multiple regional nodal basins and aberrant drainage patterns, including the head and neck or midtruncal regions.[66]

SUMMARY

Performing SLNB provides important prognostic information of thin, intermediate, and thick melanomas, allowing identification of candidates who may benefit from CLND, adjuvant therapy, clinical trial, or even observation with serial ultrasonography. Patients with intermediate-thickness melanoma who are offered and have an SLNB have been shown to have increases in both MSS and distant DFS. Although this has not been shown consistently in thin or thick melanoma, SLNB should be discussed and offered to this group because the information obtained from the biopsy seems to help direct future therapy, with a CLND, adjuvant treatment, or clinical trial. Newer radioactive tracers and overlapping imaging modalities, such as [^{99m}Tc]tilmanocept and SPET/CT, are being studied and have been shown to improve accuracy in locating and removing the SLN.

REFERENCES

1. Siegel R, Naishadham D, Jemal A. Cancer statistics, 2013. CA Cancer J Clin 2012;62:10–29.
2. Thompson JF, Shaw HM. Sentinel node mapping for melanoma: results of trials and current applications. Surg Oncol Clin N Am 2007;16:35–54.
3. Wong SL, Balch CM, Hurley P, et al. Sentinel lymph node biopsy for melanoma: American Society of Clinical Oncology and Society of Surgical Oncology Joint Clinical Practice Guideline. J Clin Oncol 2012;30(23):2912–8.
4. NCCN clinical practice guidelines in oncology (NCCN Guidelines): melanoma, version 1.2013. Fort Washington (PA): National Comprehensive Cancer Network; 2013. Available at: www.NCCN.org.
5. Reintgen D, Pendas S, Jakub J, et al. National trials involving lymphatic mapping for melanoma: the Multicenter Selective Lymphadenectomy Trial, the Sunbelt Melanoma Trial, and the Florida Melanoma Trial. Semin Oncol 2004;31:363–73.

6. Morton DL. Overview and update of the phase III Multicenter Selective Lympha-denectomy Trials (MSLT-I and MSLT-II) in melanoma. Clin Exp Metastasis 2012; 29(7):699–706.

7. Morton DL, Thompson JF, Cochran AJ, et al. Final trial report of sentinel-node bi-opsy versus nodal observation in melanoma. N Engl J Med 2014;370:599–609.

8. Morton DL, Cochran AJ. The case for lymphatic mapping and sentinel lymphade-nectomy in the management of primary melanoma. Br J Dermatol 2004;151: 308–19.

9. Thompson JF, McCarthy WH, Bosch CM, et al. Sentinel lymph node status as an indicator of the presence of metastatic melanoma in regional lymph nodes. Mel-anoma Res 1995;5:255–60.

10. Morton DL, Thompson JF, Cochran AJ, et al. Sentinel-node biopsy or nodal obser-vation in melanoma. N Engl J Med 2006;355:1307–17.

11. McMasters KM, Ross MI, Reintgen DS, et al. Final results of the Sunbelt trial. J Clin Oncol 2008;26(Suppl 15):15s [abstract: 9003].

12. McMasters KM, Noyes RD, Reintgen DS, et al. Lessons learned from the Sunbelt Melanoma Trial. J Surg Oncol 2004;86:212–23.

13. Gershenwald JE, Andtbacka RH, Prieto VG, et al. Microscopic tumor burden in sentinel lymph nodes predicts synchronous nonsentinel lymph node involvement in patients with melanoma. J Clin Oncol 2008;26:4296–303.

14. Vuylsteke RJ, Borgstein PJ, van Leeuwen PA, et al. Sentinel lymph node tumor load: an independent predictor of additional lymph node involvement and sur-vival in melanoma. Ann Surg Oncol 2005;12:440–8.

15. Veronesi U, Adamus J, Bandiera DC, et al. Inefficacy of immediate node dissec-tion in stage I melanoma of the limbs. N Engl J Med 1977;297:627–31.

16. Sim FH, Taylor WF, Pritchard DJ, et al. Lymphadenectomy in the management of stage I malignant melanoma: a prospective randomized study. Mayo Clin Proc 1986;61:697–701.

17. Cochran AJ, Wen DR, Huang RR, et al. Prediction of metastatic melanoma in non-sentinel nodes and clinical outcome based on the primary melanoma and the sentinel node. Mod Pathol 2004;17:747–55.

18. Morton DL, Cochran AJ, Thompson JF, et al. Sentinel node biopsy for early-stage melanoma: accuracy and morbidity in MSLT-I, an international multicenter trial. Ann Surg 2005;242:302–11 [discussion: 311–3].

19. Baas PC, Koops HS, Hoekstra HJ, et al. Groin dissection in the treatment of lower-extremity melanoma. Short-term and long-term morbidity. Arch Surg 1992;127: 281–6.

20. Lee JH, Essner R, Torisu-Itakura H, et al. Factors predictive of tumor-positive non-sentinel lymph nodes after tumor-positive sentinel lymph node dissection for mel-anoma. J Clin Oncol 2004;22:3677–84.

21. Han D, Zager JS, Shyr Y, et al. Clinicopathologic predictors of sentinel lymph node metastasis in thin melanoma. J Clin Oncol 2013;31:4387–93.

22. Coit DG, Andtbacka R, Anker CJ, et al. Melanoma. J Natl Compr Canc Netw 2012;10:366–400.

23. Faries MB, Wanek LA, Elashoff D, et al. Predictors of occult nodal metastasis in patients with thin melanoma. Arch Surg 2010;145:137–42.

24. Karakousis GC, Gimotty PA, Botbyl JD, et al. Predictors or regional nodal disease in patients with thin melanomas. Ann Surg Oncol 2006;13:533–41.

25. Gimotty PA, Guerry D, Ming ME, et al. Thin primary cutaneous malignant mela-noma: a prognostic tree for 10-year metastasis is more accurate than American Joint Committee on Cancer staging. J Clin Oncol 2004;22:3668–76.

26. McKinnon JG, Yu XQ, McCarthy WH, et al. Prognosis for patients with thin cutaneous melanoma: long-term survival data from New South Wales Central Cancer Registry and the Sydney Melanoma Unit. Cancer 2003;98:1223–31.

27. Balch CM, Gershenwald JE, Soong S, et al. Final version of 2009 AJCC melanoma staging and classification. J Clin Oncol 2009;27(36):6199–206.

28. Han D, Yu D, Zhao X, et al. Sentinel node biopsy is indicated for thin melanomas $\geq$ 0.76 mm. Ann Surg Oncol 2012;19(11):3335–42.

29. Kesmodel SB, Karakousis GC, Botbyl JD, et al. Mitotic rate as a predictor of sentinel lymph node positivity in patients with thin melanomas. Ann Surg Oncol 2005;12:449–58.

30. Ranieri JM, Wagner JD, Wenck S, et al. The prognostic importance of sentinel lymph node biopsy in thin melanoma. Ann Surg Oncol 2006;13:927–32.

31. Sondak VK, Taylor JM, Sabel MS, et al. Mitotic rate and younger age are predictors of sentinel lymph node positivity: lessons learned from the generation of a probabilistic model. Ann Surg Oncol 2004;11:247–58.

32. Oliveira Filho RS, Ferreira LM, Biasi LJ, et al. Vertical growth phase and positive sentinel node in thin melanoma. Braz J Med Biol Res 2003;36:347–50.

33. Bleicher RJ, Essner R, Foshag LJ, et al. Role of sentinel lymphadenectomy in thin invasive cutaneous melanomas. J Clin Oncol 2003;21:1326–31.

34. Stitzenberg KB, Groben PA, Stern SL, et al. Indications for lymphatic mapping and sentinel lymphadenectomy in patients with thin melanoma (Breslow thickness $\leq$ 1.0 mm). Ann Surg Oncol 2004;11:900–6.

35. Zettersten E, Sagebiel RW, Miller JR, et al. Prognostic factors in patients with thick cutaneous melanoma (>4 mm). Cancer 2002;94:1049–56.

36. Gershenwald JE, Mansfield PF, Lee JE, et al. Role for lymphatic mapping and sentinel lymph node biopsy in patients with thick (or $\geq$ 4 mm) primary melanoma. Ann Surg Oncol 2000;7:160–5.

37. Cherpelis BS, Haddad F, Messina J, et al. Sentinel lymph node micrometastasis and other histologic factors that predict outcome in patients with thicker melanomas. J Am Acad Dermatol 2001;44:762–6.

38. Han D, Zager JS, Yu D, et al. Desmoplastic melanoma: is there a role for sentinel lymph node biopsy? Ann Surg Oncol 2013;20(7):2345–51.

39. Busam KJ, Mujumdar U, Hummer AJ, et al. Cutaneous desmoplastic melanoma: reappraisal of morphologic heterogeneity and prognostic factors. Am J Surg Pathol 2004;28:1518–25.

40. Jaroszewski DE, Pockaj BA, DiCaudo DJ, et al. The clinical behavior of desmoplastic melanoma. Am J Surg 2001;182:590–5.

41. Livestro DP, Muzikansky A, Kaine EM, et al. Biology of desmoplastic melanoma: a case-control comparison with other melanomas. J Clin Oncol 2005;23: 6739–46.

42. Hawkins WG, Busam KJ, Ben-Porat L, et al. Desmoplastic melanoma: a pathologically and clinically distinct form of cutaneous melanoma. Ann Surg Oncol 2005; 12:207–13.

43. Pawlik TM, Ross MI, Prieto VG, et al. Assessment of the role of sentinel lymph node biopsy for primary cutaneous melanoma. Ann Surg Oncol 2005;12: 207–13.

44. Murali R, Shaw HM, Lai K, et al. Prognostic factors in cutaneous desmoplastic melanoma: a study of 252 patients. Cancer 2010;116:4130–8.

45. George E, McClain SE, Slingluff CL, et al. Subclassification of desmoplastic melanoma: pure and mixed variants have significantly different capacities for lymph node metastasis. J Cutan Pathol 2009;36:425–32.

46. Beasley GM, Speicher P, Sharma K, et al. Efficacy of repeat sentinel lymph node biopsy in patients who develop recurrent melanoma. J Am Coll Surg 2014;218: 686–92.

47. van Poll D, Thompson JF, McKinnon JG, et al. A sentinel node biopsy procedure does not increase the incidence of in-transit recurrence in patients with primary melanoma. Ann Surg Oncol 2005;12:597–608.

48. McCarthy JG, Haagensen CD, Herter FP. The role of groin dissection in the management of melanoma of the lower extremity. Ann Surg 1974;179:156–9.

49. Karakousis CP, Choe KJ, Holyoke ED. Biologic behavior and treatment of intransit metastasis of melanoma. Surg Gynecol Obstet 1980;150:29–32.

50. Cascinelli N, Bufalino R, Marolda R, et al. Regional non-nodal metastases of cutaneous melanoma. Eur J Surg Oncol 1986;12:175–80.

51. Singletary SE, Tucker SL, Boddie AW Jr. Multivariate analysis of prognostic factors in regional cutaneous metastases of extremity melanoma. Cancer 1988;61: 1437–40.

52. Coventry BJ, Chatterton B, Whitehead F, et al. Sentinel lymph node dissection and lymphatic mapping for local subcutaneous recurrence in melanoma treatment: longer-term follow-up results. Ann Surg Oncol 2004;11(3 Suppl): 203S–7S.

53. Sondak VK, King DW, Zager JS, et al. Combined analysis of phase III trials evaluating [^{99m}Tc]tilmanocept and vital blue dye for identification of sentinel lymph nodes in clinically node-negative cutaneous melanoma. Ann Surg Oncol 2013; 20(2):680–8.

54. Liu Y, Truini C, Ariyan S. A randomized study comparing the effectiveness of methylene blue dye with lymphazurin blue dye in sentinel lymph node biopsy for the treatment of cutaneous melanoma. Ann Surg Oncol 2008;15:2412–7.

55. Neves RI, Reynolds BQ, Hazard SW, et al. Increased post-operative complications with methylene blue versus lymphazurin in sentinel lymph node biopsies for skin cancers. J Surg Oncol 2011;103:421–5.

56. Liu LC, Parrett BM, Jenkins T, et al. Selective sentinel lymph node dissection for melanoma: importance of harvesting nodes with lower radioactive counts without the need for blue dye. Ann Surg Oncol 2011;18:2919–24.

57. Puleo CA, Berman C, Montilla-Soler JL, et al. 99m Tc-Tilmanocept for lymphoscintigraphy. Imag Med 2013;5(2):119–25.

58. Wallace AM, Hoh CK, Schulteis G, et al. Lymphoseek: a molecular radiopharmaceutical for sentinel node detection. Ann Surg Oncol 2003;10:531–8.

59. Wallace AM, Hoh CK, Vera DR, et al. Lymphoseek: a molecular imaging agent for melanoma sentinel lymph node mapping. Ann Surg Oncol 2007;14: 913–21.

60. van Der Ploeg IC, Olmos RR, Kroon BR, et al. The yield of SPECT/CT for anatomical lymphatic mapping in patients with melanoma. Ann Surg Oncol 2009;16:1537–42.

61. Even-Sapir E, Lerma H, Lievshitz G, et al. Lymphoscintigraphy for sentinel node mapping using a hybrid SPECT/CT system. J Nucl Med 2003;44:1413–20.

62. Vermeeren L, Valdes R, Klop M, et al. SPECT/CT for sentinel lymph node mapping in head and neck melanoma. Head Neck 2011;33(1):1–6.

63. de Wilt JH, Thompson JF, Uren RF, et al. Correlation between preoperative lymphoscintigraphy and metastatic nodal disease sites in 362 patients with cutaneous melanomas of the head and neck. Ann Surg 2004;239:544–52.

64. Carlson GW, Page AJ, Cohen C, et al. Regional recurrence after negative sentinel lymph node biopsy for melanoma. Ann Surg 2008;248:378–86.

65. Chao C, Wong SL, Edwards MJ, et al. Sentinel lymph node biopsy for head and neck melanomas. Ann Surg Oncol 2003;10:21–6.
66. Yamamoto M, Djulbegovic M, Montilla-Soler J, et al. Single photon emission computed tomography (SPECT) compared with conventional planar lymphoscintigraphy (LS) for preoperative sentinel node localization in cutaneous malignancies. Ann Surg Oncol 2013;20:233.

Lymph Node Dissection for Stage III Melanoma

Maggie L. Diller, MD, Benjamin M. Martin, MD, Keith A. Delman, MD*

KEYWORDS

- Stage III melanoma • Lymphadenectomy • Locoregional spread
- Videoscopic inguinal lymphadenectomy

KEY POINTS

- Stage III melanoma necessitates surgical intervention via complete dissection of the affected lymph node basin.
- Patients with stage III disease can be divided into 2 categories: those with microscopic disease and those with macroscopic disease.
- The surgical approach to lymphadenectomy for sentinel lymph node–positive (microscopic) or clinically palpable (macroscopic) nodal disease varies depending on the site.
- Videoscopic inguinofemoral lymphadenectomy offers a new approach to traditional groin dissection with an improved morbidity profile and maintains acceptable short-term oncologic outcomes.

INTRODUCTION

Cutaneous melanoma continues to present a considerable health problem in the United States. According to data collected by the US Centers for Disease Control and Prevention, more than 76,000 people in the United States were estimated to develop melanoma of the skin and more than 9000 people were expected to die from melanoma in 2014.[1] However, the incidence of this disease continues to increase rapidly for both genders.[1] Although research is underway to improve systemic therapies and several new treatment options have been approved for use, the prognosis for metastatic disease remains poor, with a 5-year survival of less than 20%.[1]

Nodal status is the strongest single prognostic factor in patients with melanoma.[2] The mainstay of treatment of node-positive (stage III) disease is surgical intervention

Disclosure: The authors have nothing to disclose.
Division of Surgical Oncology, Department of Surgery, Winship Cancer Institute-Emory University, 1365 Clifton Road, Atlanta, GA 30322, USA
* Corresponding author. Division of Surgical Oncology, Department of Surgery, Winship Cancer Institute-Emory University School of Medicine, 1365 Clifton Road, Northeast Suite C2004, Atlanta, GA 30322.
E-mail address: kdelman@emory.edu

via complete dissection of the affected lymph node basin. In the era of sentinel lymph node biopsy (SLNB), patients with occult disease are detected early, and there is evidence that shows a benefit to immediate completion lymphadenectomy with improved disease-free and melanoma-specific survival.[3] Despite these data, a recent assessment of the quality of cancer care in the United States indicates that close to 50% of patients with positive nodes do not undergo appropriate surgical intervention, likely secondary to concerns about potential morbidity of lymphadenectomy.[4] With the incidence of melanoma continuing to increase, new systemic therapeutic options, and improved diagnostic and staging techniques, a complete understanding of the surgical approach to stage III melanoma is paramount.

PATIENT EVALUATION OVERVIEW

Stage III melanoma is locoregional disease. It is characterized by nodal disease, local recurrence, or in-transit disease. This article focuses solely on nodal disease. In assessing treatment strategies, patients with stage III disease can be divided into 2 categories: those with microscopic disease and those with macroscopic disease.

Microscopic Disease

Indications and approach to SLNB are covered in detail elsewhere in this issue. Data have shown that 16% to 20% of patients with a positive SLNB harbor additional positive lymph nodes[5,6] and are at greater risk for disseminated disease.[7] Current practice is to perform completion lymph node dissection (CLND) in patients with a positive SLNB; this practice is supported by the MSLT-1 trial that showed improved 10-year disease-free survival rates in patients undergoing immediate versus delayed lymphadenectomy.[3]

Patients with microscopic disease do not warrant preoperative imaging unless symptomatic because routine radiographic staging rarely yields significant information.[8,9] In addition, in the setting of microscopic disease, anatomic considerations are almost uniformly negligible, and therefore imaging to assess resectability in this patient population is not indicated. As these patients have likely been evaluated for general anesthesia previously, they do not require additional preoperative testing.

Macroscopic Disease

Individuals with palpable nodal disease carry a significantly worse prognosis than those with microscopic disease.[10] Confirmation of metastatic disease in patients with clinical or radiographically identified lymphadenopathy should be obtained with fine-needle aspiration biopsy (FNA). FNA is preferred rather than excisional biopsy for histologic confirmation of disease before surgical intervention, although there is conflicting evidence regarding regional control with lymphadenectomy after FNA in contrast with excision.[11,12] In patients with macroscopic disease, staging evaluation (computed tomography [CT], PET/CT, MRI) is advocated before intervening surgically in order to identify those people who might harbor occult metastatic disease and in whom surgical control of regional disease has only a limited role.

Preoperative considerations for patients intended to undergo completion lymphadenectomy include physiologic and anatomic concerns. As with all procedures, ability to tolerate general anesthesia remains paramount. Although some experts consider performing lymphadenectomies under sedation or regional anesthesia, the authors of this article do not find that a feasible approach and exclusively use general anesthesia. In addition, it is very unusual for lymphatic metastases without prior treatment to be inseparable from major neurovascular structures. Given this, it is rare that volume of disease proves prohibitive to surgical resection. Nonetheless, extent of disease and proximity to or involvement of neurovascular structures should be considered on preoperative evaluation.

In the absence of a clinical trial for neoadjuvant systemic therapy, and with histologic confirmation and no evidence of distant metastases, surgical intervention is recommended. The specific procedure performed depends on the site and extent of disease, which is detailed in later sections.

NONSURGICAL TREATMENT OPTIONS

The following means of therapy (neoadjuvant/adjuvant, radiation, and so forth) are discussed in detail elsewhere in this issue. This article limits the discussion of these modalities to their context in the setting of surgical lymphadenectomy.

Pharmacologic Treatment Options: Neoadjuvant and Adjuvant Therapy

Patients at high risk of recurrence following surgical treatment are candidates for adjuvant therapy. Both high-dose interferon alfa-2b (HDI) and pegylated interferon, characterized by a longer half-life, are approved for the adjuvant treatment of patients at high risk for relapse. Randomized controlled trials have identified bulky lymph node disease as well as ulceration of the primary tumor as independent predictors for benefit from adjuvant interferon.[13] HDI and pegylated interferon alfa-2b are associated with improved relapse-free survival in patients with stage II and III melanoma compared with low-dose interferon or observation alone.[14,15] Despite statistical significance, many specialists are still hesitant to use interferon, particularly in older patients, because the response rate is modest and side effects are significant.

The use of neoadjuvant therapy is gaining popularity as understanding of tumor biology improves. One study used HDI in patients with bulky lymphadenopathy (stage IIIb–c) to enhance surgical resectability and minimize risk of relapse.[16] Advances in immunomodulation and targeted therapies have improved systemic treatment of disseminated disease and are being studied in both the adjuvant and neoadjuvant settings.[17] Monoclonal antibodies targeting extracellular T-cell receptors programmed cell death 1 (PD-1) and cytotoxic T-lymphocyte-associated protein 4 (CTLA4) as well as those targeting intracellular pathways such as BRAF inhibitors and mitogen activated protein kinase (MEK) inhibitors have gained much attention given their success in the treatment of advanced metastatic disease.

Nonpharmacologic Treatment Options: Radiation Therapy

Recent data published from randomized clinical trials indicate a role for adjuvant radiotherapy in the treatment of melanoma.[18,19] Patients with bulky lymphadenopathy and features correlating with high risk of recurrence are most likely to benefit. Although several studies report reduction in lymph node field relapse in patients receiving radiation therapy after complete lymphadenectomy, there is no clear survival benefit.[18,20] Additional information regarding the long-term morbidities associated with radiotherapy and quality-of-life outcomes is being collected; however, given these uncertainties, many clinicians are still cautious regarding its use.

Combination Therapies

With the introduction of new immunotherapies targeting specific cell receptors and intracellular pathways, optimizing combinations of these medications could lead to major improvements in medical management. For example, ipilimumab, an anti-CTLA4 antibody, has recently been combined with pembrolizumab, an anti-PD1 antibody, with tumor regression rates greater than 80% in most responders.[21] As the treatments for disseminated disease evolve, their use can be studied in both the neo-adjuvant and adjuvant settings, maximizing surgical control.

SURGICAL TREATMENT OPTIONS AND TECHNIQUE

Surgical therapy is the mainstay of treatment of patients with positive lymph nodes, whether detected by SLNB, imaging, or clinical examination. For patients with regional disease identified via SLNB, completion lymphadenectomy of the involved basin is performed. Patients with clinically palpable nodes also undergo lymphadenectomy, alternatively termed therapeutic lymphadenectomy.

Note that, in the setting of microscopic disease, lymph node basins should be managed based on the sentinel node status of that particular basin.[22] Involved regional basins amenable to surgical intervention include cervical, axillary, inguinal, pelvic (iliac), and less commonly the epitrochlear or popliteal nodal basins, which is particularly important in patients with drainage to multiple basins or in those with unusual drainage patterns. Occasionally, lymphoscintigraphy identifies an aberrant or interval lymph node basin outside the typical regions listed earlier. Although the management of these lymph nodes is discussed later, appropriate biopsy is imperative at the time of the initial SLNB.[22]

Cervical Lymphadenectomy

Cervical lymph node basins can harbor metastases from the head and neck, the upper trunk, and occasionally from an unknown primary site. In general, a modified neck dissection including levels II, III, IV, and V (sparing the spinal accessory nerve, the sternocleidomastoid muscle (SCM), and the internal jugular vein) is the procedure of choice in patients with positive lymph node basins in this region. Patients with drainage through the parotid gland, with nodes identified in the parotid, and those with tumors on the frontal scalp and temporal areas should undergo concurrent superficial parotidectomy. According to validated melanoma quality indicators, a patient undergoing cervical lymphadenectomy with involvement of 4 or more levels should have at least 20 nodes resected and evaluated.[18,23] Radical neck dissections are reserved for patients showing direct tumor extension to one of these structures. In patients with microscopic disease, there may be a role for selective neck dissection (involving even fewer anatomic regions), although evidence supporting this remains lacking.[24]

Incisions for neck dissection can be oriented in a variety of ways. For a posterolateral dissection, an L-shaped incision allows better visualization of the 11th cranial nerve and level V lymph nodes.[24] The incision runs along the anterior aspect of the sternocleidomastoid and curves laterally along the clavicle, thus forming an L shape; when needed, an anterior extension may be performed to create an inverted T (**Fig. 1**). The procedure can be simplified into the following steps:

- The external jugular vein is identified and divided near the upper limits of dissection, along the sternocleidomastoid muscle.
- The external jugular vein and all associated lymph nodes and fatty tissue are dissected free in a cephalad to caudad manner.
- The sternocleidomastoid is then elevated and fatty and lymphatic tissue is dissected off the internal jugular vein, also moving cephalad to caudad.
- At the anterior border of the sternocleidomastoid, the omohyoid is divided as it crosses the jugular vein.
- Dissection is carried to the base of the neck and the surgical specimen is carefully separated from the posterior aspect of the clavicle.

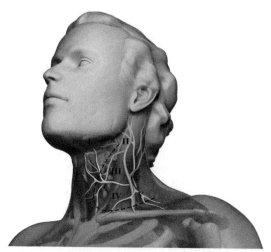

Fig. 1. Incision for cervical lymphadenectomy and lymph node levels. (*From* Delman KA, Mansfield PF, Lee JE. Indications and techniques of regional lymphadenectomy. In: Pollock RE, Curley SA, Ross MI, et al, editors. Advanced therapy in surgical oncology. Shelton (CT): PMPH; 2007. p. 771–82; with permission.)

- The external jugular vein is divided inferiorly and the omohyoid divided laterally, and the operative specimen is removed en bloc.
- For deep dissection, the deep cervical fascia is identified. Fatty and lymphatic tissue just above this fascia is removed, moving in a caudad to cephalad direction.
- Cranial nerve XI is skeletonized to its most proximal extent behind the apex of the sternocleidomastoid.
- In general, transverse cervical nerve roots are sacrificed, leaving only a sensory deficit for the patient.

Once the specimen has been removed, it is necessary to ensure hemostasis. The patient is often placed in Trendelenburg position and a Valsalva maneuver is implemented. In the case of significant dissection, lymphatic leaks may be evident and suture ligation of individual lymphatics is necessary. Although in recent years the advent of a multitude of different energy devices has prompted consideration of newer devices, potentially reducing the incidence of lymphatic leakage, this has not been borne out in any analysis to date. Topical sealants have not been shown to reduce the incidence of lymphatic leak either.[25] The sternal head of the sternocleidomastoid may be mobilized and placed over leaky tributaries, if desired. In addition, a closed suction drain should be placed within the surgical bed.

Disease occasionally extends into the central neck, mediastinum, or below the clavicle, and this is evident via imaging or intraoperative findings. The presence of pathologically involved lymph nodes should direct the extent of surgery.

In general, hospital stay after cervical lymphadenectomy is brief, with patients discharged home on postoperative day 1. Patients should be given a diet before discharge in order to assess drain output for chyle. In the presence of high-volume lymphatic leaks (>200 mL per day), immediate surgical intervention with ligation of the involved lymphatic tributaries is recommended.[24] For low-volume lymphatic leaks, patients can be placed on fat-restricted diets and drain output monitored. Drains are left in place until daily output is less than 15 mL, which is usually within 1 week.

Axillary Lymphadenectomy

A complete axillary dissection of levels I, II, and III with resection and evaluation of at least 20 nodes is routinely performed for melanoma.[23,24] In an era when extent of surgery is being questioned, and in which as many as 80% of patients with sentinel lymph node–detected disease do not have additional disease at completion lymphadenectomy, at least 1 recent study has called into question the need for a level III dissection.[26] Until additional data regarding this are available or MSLT-2 reaches maturity, the standard recommendations remain for complete dissection.

A lazy-S incision is used, beginning along the edge of the pectoralis major muscle and extending downward across the axilla. The incision continues inferiorly along the anterior border of the latissimus dorsi muscle. The dissection extends superiorly to the tendinous portion of the pectoralis major and inferiorly to the junction of the latissimus and serratus muscles. The steps of dissection are as follows:

- Fascia along the lateral aspect of the latissimus is mobilized and dissection proceeds up to the insertion of this muscle, protecting the thoracodorsal neurovascular bundle lying inferiorly.
- Fascia of the pectoralis major is mobilized and dissection performed posteriorly, accessing those nodes between the pectoralis major and minor (Rotter nodes) **Fig. 2**.
- Tissue between these two muscles is swept laterally into the axilla.
- Dissection of the inferior portion of the wound begins and tissue from the serratus anterior muscle is mobilized, anterior to the subscapularis, offering visualization of the thoracodorsal neurovascular bundle.
- The long thoracic nerve is also identified and the surgical specimen is dissected away from both nerve bundles, up to the level of the axillary vein.
- The axillary vein is skeletonized from a lateral to medial approach and tissue superficial and superior to the axillary vein is swept into the axilla.
  - This part of the operation takes place directly above the brachial plexus. Flexion of the elbow and shoulder is often helpful, offering access to the deepest portions of the axilla.[24]
- The pectoralis minor is then elevated, offering visualization of the medial portion of the axillary vein. Retraction of the pectoralis musculature is best achieved via an assistant on the contralateral side of the table. Alternatively, division of the pectoralis minor may be necessary to access the level III nodes.
- Remaining tissue is dissected free in a lateral to medial fashion up to the level of the Halsted ligament, which is a condensation of clavipectoral fascia (**Fig. 3**).

Once this portion of the procedure has concluded, the specimen can be removed from the axilla. A closed suction drain should be left in the wound bed, completing the surgery.

Postoperative care is generally straightforward with the patient discharged home the following day, although some surgeons send patients home the same day. Drain output should be less than 30 mL per day before removal. Ideally, drains are removed within 21 days of surgery.

Inguinofemoral (Superficial) and Ilioinguinal (Deep) Lymphadenectomy

Depending on the extent of disease, patients with inguinal lymphadenopathy undergo either superficial groin dissection (inguinofemoral dissection) or a superficial and deep

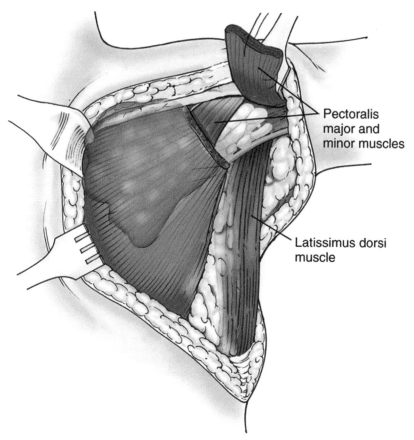

Fig. 2. Division of the fascia of the pectoralis major allows access to the Rotter nodes. (*From* Wobbes T, Hoekstra HJJ. Composite axillary and supraclavicular lymph node dissection. In: Khatri VP, editor. Atlas of advanced operative surgery. Philadelphia: Elsevier; 2013. p. 494–9; with permission.)

dissection (ilioinguinal dissection). In patients with microscopic disease and less than 4 involved nodes, and without intraoperative findings to indicate clinically positive disease, most surgeons biopsy the Cloquet node. This node lies just within the pelvis, slightly posterior and medial to the external iliac vein. As such, patients undergoing a superficial groin dissection should be prepped to allow extension to a deep dissection should intraoperative findings indicate necessity. Per validated quality indicators, at least 7 lymph nodes should be removed and evaluated during an inguinal dissection.[23] However, the authors do not routinely biopsy the Cloquet node, using data from 2 studies performed at Emory University Hospital to modify practice.[27] In current practice, a superficial inguinal lymphadenectomy only is performed in patients with stage IIIA disease.

A longitudinal, lazy-S incision is made, beginning superior and medial to the anterior superior iliac spine and running parallel within the groin crease, extending vertically down the leg to the apex of the femoral triangle (**Fig. 4**B). The steps for performing a superficial dissection are discussed later.

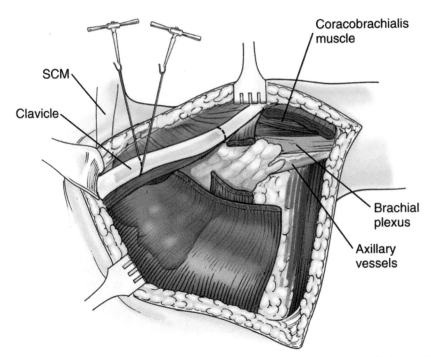

Fig. 3. Retraction or division of the pectoralis minor offers visualization of the medial portion of the axillary vein and access to level III nodes. SCM, sternocleidomastoid muscle. (*From* Wobbes T, Hoekstra HJJ. Composite axillary and supraclavicular lymph node dissection. In: Khatri VP, editor. Atlas of advanced operative surgery. Philadelphia: Elsevier; 2013. p. 494–9; with permission.)

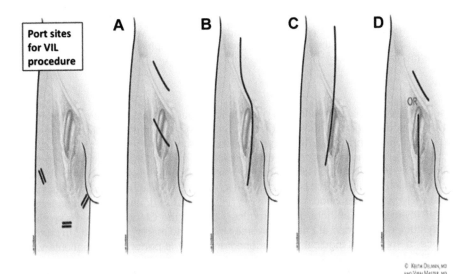

Fig. 4. Incisions for groin dissection. The image at far left depicts port placement for videoscopic inguinal lymphadenectomy (VIL). (*A-D*) Variations used during open technique. (*From* Keith A. Delman, Atlanta (GA); with permission.)

Superficial Dissection

- Lymph node–bearing tissue overlying the external oblique aponeurosis is swept from approximately 5 cm above the inguinal ligament inferiorly into the femoral triangle.
- Tissue overlying the lateral portion of the sartorius is mobilized, including the fascia.
  - The femoral nerve runs along the medial portion of this same muscle and is identified and preserved.
- At the apex of the femoral triangle, tissue is dissected in an inferior to superior manner (**Fig. 5**).
- Medially, the dissection extends along the adductor longus, excluding the fascia.
- The saphenous vein is identified crossing the adductor longus muscle. It can be ligated along with the many lymphatics present in this area.
  - In pediatric patients or patients with truncal lesions, the saphenous vein can be preserved and may result in decreased lower-extremity edema.[24] However, it is imperative that the lymph node–containing tissue be completely dissected away from the saphenous vein and removed.
- The anterior surface of the femoral artery is skeletonized.
- The dissection continues medially and posteriorly, skeletonizing the femoral vein.
- The specimen is dissected away from the vessels superiorly to the level of the saphenofemoral junction. The saphenous vein is divided at this level.
- The lymphatics over the medial aspect of the femoral vein represent the only remaining attachments and are ligated at the level of the femoral canal, allowing removal of the surgical specimen.

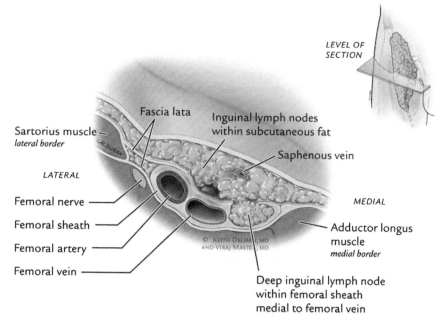

Fig. 5. Cross-sectional view of the femoral triangle. (*From* Keith A. Delman, Atlanta (GA); with permission.)

At this point in the surgery, if the surgeon chooses to, biopsy of the Cloquet node is performed. In order to do so, the surgeon creates a femoral hernia by incising the lacunar ligament. The sampled node is then sent for frozen section and the wound irrigated and packed until the decision to close versus proceed with a deep dissection is made.

Deep Pelvic Dissection

A deep pelvic dissection should be performed in the following patient populations: (1) those with microscopic disease but involvement of 4 or more nodes, (2) palpable lymph nodes, (3) a positive Cloquet node, or (4) cross-sectional imaging suggesting deep ilioinguinal nodal disease. The steps for a deep dissection are as follows:

- Skin incision is extended superiorly over the abdominal wall and the underlying muscles are divided in the direction of the fibers of the external oblique. The peritoneum is mobilized and retracted medially, exposing the retroperitoneum.
- The ureter is identified and protected and the inferior epigastric vessels retracted or ligated.
- External iliac vessels are visualized, and skeletonized up to the bifurcation of the common iliac vessels.
- Grossly positive nodal disease proximal to the common iliac bifurcation can be removed; however, this portends a poor prognosis and classifies a patient as stage IV.
- The next step involves blunt dissection of the obturator nodes, carefully identifying and sparing the obturator nerve and vessels.
- Unless grossly positive, nodal tissue posterior to the obturator nerve is left in place to avoid damaging this structure.[24]
- The obturator lymph nodes represent the third nodal specimen sent to pathology.
- Nodal packets are sent and evaluated separately such that pathologists can characterize the extent of disease of each distinct compartment.[24]

A drain is placed solely in the superficial groin. The femoral canal should be closed. In all cases, use of a sartorius muscle flap to cover the femoral vessels is recommended.[24] Given that most series report the incidence of wound complications from this procedure to be very high, this offers protection to the underlying vasculature should the wound break down.

Patients undergoing superficial dissection are usually discharged home the following day. Although this may take considerably longer, we prefer to remove all drains by postoperative day 21. In patients undergoing sartorius muscle transposition, bed rest is often recommended for the first 24 hours.[24]

Modifications of Open Superficial Inguinal Lymphadenectomy

Given the high morbidity attributed to open inguinal lymphadenectomy, considerable effort has been made to reduce the risk of complications from this procedure. Alternative approaches include modifying the choice of incision (see **Fig. 4**A, C, D), sparing the saphenous vein, and limiting the extent of the dissection based on the location of the primary lesion (abdominal wall lesions would include dissection of the upper groin, whereas lower-extremity lesions would include dissection of the lower groin, with both including the saphenofemoral junction). The authors modified a procedure originally described by Tobias-Machado and colleagues[28] for genitourinary malignancies and examined a videoscopic approach to inguinofemoral lymphadenectomy (**Fig. 6**). This procedure has shown equal pathologic and short-term

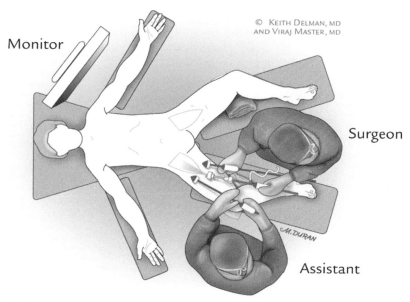

© Keith Delman, MD
and Viraj Master, MD

Monitor

Surgeon

Assistant

Fig. 6. Patient and surgeon positioning for video-assisted lymphadenectomy. (*From* Martin BM, Master VA, Delman KA. Minimizing morbidity in melanoma surgery. Oncology (Williston Park) 2013;27(10):1016–20; with permission.)

oncologic outcomes with a marked reduction in complications.[29] The procedure is as follows:

- An apical port is placed 3 cm inferior to the apex of the femoral triangle (see **Fig. 4**).
- Flaps are raised in the standard plane of dissection, just superficial to the continuation of the Scarpa fascia to the planned working ports.
- Two additional working ports are placed 2 cm lateral and medial to the boundaries of the femoral triangle at the level of the apex.
- The remainder of the flap is raised to the level of the complete dissection, 5 cm above the inguinal ligament.
- All of the inguinal contents are then dissected, skeletonizing the femoral vasculature and removing all of the fibrofatty tissue in the inguinofemoral region.

This procedure is described in additional detail elsewhere[29] and should only be performed either on protocol or by someone who is comfortable performing an open inguinal lymphadenectomy.

Epitrochlear Lymphadenectomy

In the past, dissection of the epitrochlear and popliteal regions was uncommon. However, with the advent of lymphoscintigraphy and SLNB, dissection of these areas has increased.[24] The incision begins approximately 8 cm above and just anterior to the medial epicondyle. It extends in a slight hockey-stick fashion across the antecubital fossae for 4 to 5 cm and continues over the tendinous portion of the biceps muscle (**Fig. 7**). The steps are as follows:

- The lymph node–containing tissue is dissected off the biceps and swept into the fossa.

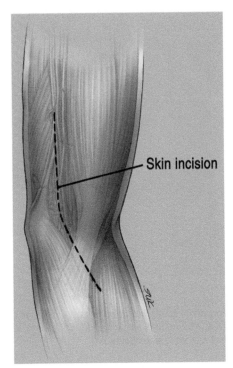

Skin incision

Fig. 7. Incision for epitrochlear dissection. (*From* Delman KA, Mansfield PF, Lee JE. Indications and techniques of regional lymphadenectomy. Pollock RE, Curley SA, Ross MI, et al, editors. Advanced therapy in surgical oncology. Shelton (CT): PMPH; 2007. p. 771–82; with permission.)

- Additional tissue between the biceps and triceps muscles is also dissected free.
- The brachial artery and vein, and median and ulnar nerves are identified and protected.
- All tissue is swept distally, freeing it from the vessels and nerves, up to the intersection of the biceps muscles and wrist flexors.
- A drain is left in place and the wound closed.

Popliteal Lymphadenectomy

In preparing for dissection of the popliteal fossa, the patient is placed in the prone position. Should an inguinal dissection also be indicated, dissection of the popliteal region is performed first. The incision takes the shape of a lazy S and begins 10 cm above the joint crease, moves transversely across the joint, and extends longitudinally down the leg for approximately 10 cm (**Fig. 8**). The incision may move from a superolateral to inferomedial direction or vice versa, depending on orientation of prior scars. The steps are as follows:

- The boundaries of the popliteal fossa are exposed, including the biceps femoris and semitendinosus muscles.
- The tibial and common peroneal nerves are visualized between these muscles and are preserved.
- The nodal tissues is swept away from these nerves and moved distally, exposing the popliteal artery and vein.

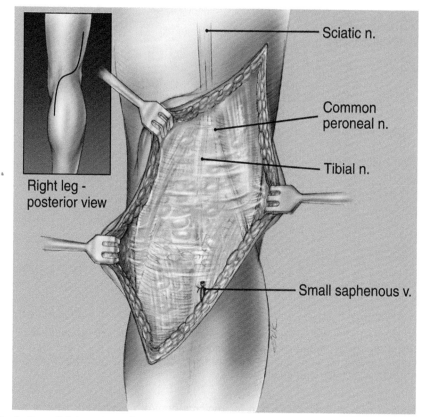

Fig. 8. Superficial exposure during popliteal dissection. n, nerve; v, vein. (*From* Delman KA, Mansfield PF, Lee JE. Indications and techniques of regional lymphadenectomy. Pollock RE, Curley SA, Ross MI, et al, editors. Advanced therapy in surgical oncology. Shelton (CT): PMPH; 2007. p. 771–82; with permission.)

- Nodal tissue surrounding the artery and vein is also dissected free.
  - It is important to include tissue lying on the far side of these vessels in order to ensure a complete dissection.[24]
- The dissection is carried distally along these vessels until they descend behind the gastrocnemius muscle (**Fig. 9**).
- The tissue is removed and a drain is placed.

TREATMENT RESISTANCE AND COMPLICATIONS

Locoregional recurrence rates in patients undergoing surgical resection with lymphadenectomy are reported at approximately 20%.[30] Rates of recurrence are similar among those with microscopic and macroscopic disease (19% vs 22%) according to a recent study.[30] Although therapeutic lymphadenectomy is the standard of care recommended by the National Comprehensive Cancer Network for patients with melanoma with node-positive disease,[31] up to 50% of these patients do not undergo completion lymphadenectomy,[4] likely in part because of the morbidity associated with regional lymphadenectomy, which varies by nodal basin.

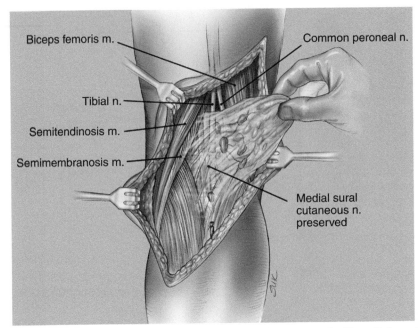

Fig. 9. Removal of nodal packet during popliteal dissection. m, muscle. (*From* Delman KA, Mansfield PF, Lee JE. Indications and techniques of regional lymphadenectomy. Pollock RE, Curley SA, Ross MI, et al, editors. Advanced therapy in surgical oncology. Shelton (CT): PMPH; 2007. p. 771–82; with permission.)

Modified radical neck dissection for regional control of involved cervical lymph nodes has been associated with complications as high as 10%.[32] Complications unique to the modified radical neck dissection include shoulder dysfunction related to injury or devascularization of the spinal accessory nerve and chyle leaks from thoracic duct injuries. Note that this is a marked improvement compared with previous rates seen with the radical neck dissection. A selective approach to cervical lymph node dissection has been advocated for patients with sentinel lymph node–positive disease, which may further limit morbidity[33] but will potentially trade off this benefit for a higher risk of in-basin recurrence.

One comprehensive study measured morbidity of completion axillary lymphadenectomy to be approximately 23%.[34] Short-term concerns include seroma formation or lymphorrhea caused by persistent lymph drainage, which predisposes to wound breakdown and infection. Loss of sensation in the upper, inner arm may occur because of sacrifice of the intercostobrachial nerve. The primary long-term concern is lymphedema, which had an incidence of 5% in the Sunbelt Melanoma Trial.[34]

Inguinal lymphadenectomy is associated with significant morbidity, as mentioned previously. Multiple studies have shown complication rates as high as 50%. Wound infection, dehiscence, seroma formation, skin flap necrosis, lymphedema, and deep vein thrombosis are all concerns. Technical modifications to the open technique, such as sartorius transposition, have not substantially decreased complications.[35] However, the application of minimally invasive technology to perform videoscopic inguinal lymphadenectomy has recently been shown to reduce morbidity and preserve equivalent oncologic outcomes. In a comprehensive analysis with an exhaustive dictionary of complications, wound-related complications were markedly reduced compared with the open technique (47.5% vs 80%, respectively).[35]

OUTCOMES AND LONG-TERM RECOMMENDATIONS

Although melanoma remains a predominantly surgically managed disease, judicious implementation of procedures is important given the associated morbidities, particularly lymphadenectomy. Ten-year follow-up data from the MSLT-I trial have recently become available. Results of the study indicate that patients with intermediate-thickness melanomas and positive SLNB who underwent immediate completion lymphadenectomy have improved disease-free, distant disease–free, and melanoma-specific survival rates compared with patients in whom lymphadenectomy was delayed until nodal relapse.[3] The investigators' final analysis indicates a tripling of disease-free survival and doubling of both melanoma-specific and distant disease–free survivals with early intervention.[3] Although there was an improved 10-year disease-free survival in patients with thick melanomas undergoing immediate lymphadenectomy versus observation (50% vs 40%), no increases in distant disease–free and melanoma-specific survival were observed.[3]

Although the MSLT-I trial concluded that early detection and removal of microscopic nodal disease improve outcomes, less than 20% of patients undergoing completion lymphadenectomy have nodal metastases outside the sentinel node.[36] The MSLT-II trial is a randomized, phase III trial that has completed accrual and is undergoing data analysis. Patients with a positive SLN were randomized 2:1 to undergo either ultrasonography surveillance or completion lymphadenectomy. The investigators hypothesize that CLND can be avoided in many patients with sentinel node metastases.[36]

SUMMARY

Surgery remains the primary therapy in patients with nodal metastases, with lymphadenectomy the standard of care. However, lymphadenectomy has complications and research is underway that is likely to change the approach to many patients. Results of the MSLT-II trial may serve to further narrow the patient population for which lymphadenectomy is recommended. The development of innovative systemic therapies holds promise in the treatment of widely disseminated disease. Conceptual understanding of melanoma continues to evolve at a rapid pace and, as clinicians and scientists improve their understanding of the pathobiology driving this disease, management strategies will continue to evolve.

REFERENCES

1. Rebecca S, Jiemin M, Zhaohui Z, et al. Cancer statistics, 2014. CA Cancer J Clin 2014;64(1):9–29.
2. Balch Charles M, Seng-Jaw S, Gershenwald Jeffrey E, et al. Prognostic factors analysis of 17,600 melanoma patients: validation of the American Joint Committee on Cancer melanoma staging system. J Clin Oncol 2001;19(16):3622–34.
3. Morton Donald L, Thompson John F, Cochran Alistair J, et al. Final trial report of sentinel-node biopsy versus nodal observation in melanoma. N Engl J Med 2014; 370(7):599–609.
4. Bilimoria KY, Balch CM, Bentrem DJ, et al. Complete lymph node dissection for sentinel node-positive melanoma: assessment of practice patterns in the United States. Ann Surg Oncol 2008;15(6):1566–76.

5. Natale C, Emilio B, Rosaria B, et al. Sentinel and nonsentinel node status in stage IB and II melanoma patients: two-step prognostic indicators of survival. J Clin Oncol 2006;24(27):4464–71.

6. Lee Jonathan H, Richard E, Hitoe T-I, et al. Factors predictive of tumor-positive nonsentinel lymph nodes after tumor-positive sentinel lymph node dissection for melanoma. J Clin Oncol 2004;22(18):3677–84.

7. Gershenwald JE, Ross MI. Sentinel-lymph-node biopsy for cutaneous melanoma. N Engl J Med 2011;364(18):1738–45.

8. Aloia TA, Gershenwald JE, Andtbacka RH, et al. Utility of computed tomography and magnetic resonance imaging staging before completion lymphadenectomy in patients with sentinel lymph node-positive melanoma. J Clin Oncol 2006; 24(18):2858–65.

9. Miranda EP, Gertner M, Wall J, et al. Routine imaging of asymptomatic melanoma patients with metastasis to sentinel lymph nodes rarely identifies systemic disease. Arch Surg 2004;139(8):831–6 [discussion: 836–7].

10. Balch CM, Soong S-J, Atkins MB, et al. An evidence-based staging system for cutaneous melanoma. CA Cancer J Clin 2004;54(3):131–49.

11. Kelemen PR, Wanek LA, Morton DL. Lymph node biopsy does not impair survival after therapeutic dissection for palpable melanoma metastases. Ann Surg Oncol 1999;6(2):139–43.

12. Morton DL, Thompson JF, Cochran AJ, et al. Sentinel-node biopsy or nodal observation in melanoma. N Engl J Med 2006;355(13):1307–17.

13. Eggermont AM, Suciu S, Testori A, et al. Ulceration and stage are predictive of interferon efficacy in melanoma: results of the phase III adjuvant trials EORTC 18952 and EORTC 18991. Eur J Cancer 2012;48(2):218–25.

14. Eggermont AM, Suciu S, Santinami M, et al. Adjuvant therapy with pegylated interferon alfa-2b versus observation alone in resected stage III melanoma: final results of EORTC 18991, a randomised phase III trial. Lancet 2008;372(9633):117–26.

15. Kirkwood JM, Ibrahim JG, Sondak VK, et al. High- and low-dose interferon alfa-2b in high-risk melanoma: first analysis of intergroup trial E1690/S9111/C9190. J Clin Oncol 2000;18(12):2444–58.

16. Tarhini AA, Pahuja S, Kirkwood JM. Neoadjuvant therapy for high-risk bulky regional melanoma. J Surg Oncol 2011;104(4):386–90.

17. La Greca M, Grasso G, Antonelli G, et al. Neoadjuvant therapy for locally advanced melanoma: new strategies with targeted therapies. Onco Targets Ther 2014;7:1115–21.

18. Burmeister BH, Henderson MA, Ainslie J, et al. Adjuvant radiotherapy versus observation alone for patients at risk of lymph-node field relapse after therapeutic lymphadenectomy for melanoma: a randomised trial. Lancet Oncol 2012;13(6): 589–97.

19. Burmeister BH, Mark Smithers B, Burmeister E, et al. A prospective phase II study of adjuvant postoperative radiation therapy following nodal surgery in malignant melanoma–Trans Tasman Radiation Oncology Group (TROG) Study 96.06. Radiother Oncol 2006;81(2):136–42.

20. Ballo MT, Ang KK. Radiation therapy for malignant melanoma. Surg Clin North Am 2003;83(2):323–42.

21. Brahmer JR, Tykodi SS, Chow LQM, et al. Safety and activity of anti–PD-L1 antibody in patients with advanced cancer. N Engl J Med 2012;366(26): 2455–65.

22. Love TP, Delman KA. Management of regional lymph node basins in melanoma. Ochsner J 2010;10(2):99–107.

23. Spillane AJ, Cheung BL, Stretch JR, et al. Proposed quality standards for regional lymph node dissections in patients with melanoma. Ann Surg 2009;249(3): 473–80.

24. Delman KA, Mansfield PF, Lee JE. Indications and techniques of regional lympha-denectomy. In: Curley SA, Pollock RE, Ross MI, editors. Advanced therapy in sur-gical oncology. Shelton (CT): PMPH; 2007. p. 771–82.

25. Mortenson MM, Xing Y, Weaver S. Fibrin sealant does not decrease seroma output or time to drain removal following inguino-femoral lymph node dissection in melanoma patients: a randomized controlled trial (NCT00506311). World J Surg Oncol 2008;6:63–71.

26. Namm JP, Chang AE, Cimmino VM, et al. Is a level III dissection necessary for a positive sentinel lymph node in melanoma? J Surg Oncol 2012;105(3):225–8.

27. Chu CK, Delman KA, Carlson GW, et al. Inguinopelvic lymphadenectomy following positive inguinal sentinel lymph node biopsy in melanoma: true fre-quency of synchronous pelvic metastases. Ann Surg Oncol 2011;18(12): 3309–15.

28. Tobias-Machado M, Tavares A, Molina WR Jr, et al. Video endoscopic inguinal lymphadenectomy (VEIL): initial case report and comparison with open radical procedure. Arch Esp Urol 2006;59(8):849–52.

29. Martin BM, Master VA, Delman KA. Videoscopic inguinal lymphadenectomy for metastatic melanoma. Cancer Control 2013;20(4):255–60.

30. Veenstra HJ, van der Ploeg IMC, Wouters MW, et al. Reevaluation of the locore-gional recurrence rate in melanoma patients with a positive sentinel node compared to patients with palpable nodal involvement. Ann Surg Oncol 2010; 17(2):521–6.

31. Coit DG, Andtbacka R, Anker CJ, et al. Melanoma, version 2.2013: featured up-dates to the NCCN guidelines. J Natl Compr Canc Netw 2013;11(4):395–407.

32. Serpell JW, Carne PW, Bailey M. Radical lymph node dissection for melanoma. ANZ J Surg 2003;73(5):294–9.

33. Robbins KT. Indications for selective neck dissection: when, how, and why. Oncology (Williston Park) 2000;14(10):1455–64 [discussion: 1467–9].

34. McMasters KM, Ross I, Reintgen DS, et al. Final results of the Sunbelt Melanoma Trial. J Clin Oncol 2008;26(15S):9003 [abstract: 9003].

35. Martin BM, Master VA, Delman KA. Minimizing morbidity in melanoma surgery. Oncology (Williston Park) 2013;27(10):1016–20.

36. Morton DL. Overview and update of the phase III multicenter selective lymphade-nectomy trials (MSLT-I and MSLT-II) in melanoma. Clin Exp Metastasis 2012;29(7): 699–706.

Metastasectomy for Stage IV Melanoma

Gary B. Deutsch, MD, Daniel D. Kirchoff, MD, Mark B. Faries, MD*

KEYWORDS

- Metastatic melanoma • Metastasectomy • Oligometastases • Stage IV melanoma
- Surgery

KEY POINTS

- Outcomes are poor for most patients with stage IV metastatic melanoma.
- Surgery provides well-selected patients with a significantly improved chance at long disease-free and overall survival.
- Surgery will continue to serve as a complement to investigational and approved immunotherapeutic and targeted approaches.

INTRODUCTION

Once it has spread to distant disease sites, melanoma is notable for its difficulty to treat and poor long-term outcomes. More than 9000 patients with cutaneous melanoma succumb to the disease each year in the United States alone.[1] Patients with stage IV disease have an estimated median overall survival of 7.5 months and a 5-year survival rate of 6%.[2]

There is no consensus for the preferred treatment of stage IV melanoma. Systemic medical therapy (SMT), as in many other stage IV cancers, has been the mainstay of treatment. However, most systemic therapies have failed to offer a durable response.[3] For many years no systemic therapy showed any benefit in survival, making them palliative options, at best. In contrast, metastasectomy in appropriate candidates was

Disclosures: Supported in part by funding from Dr Miriam & Sheldon G. Adelson Medical Research Foundation (Boston, MA), the Borstein Family Foundation (Los Angeles, CA), and National Cancer Institute grants P01 CA29605 and R01 CA189163. The content is solely the responsibility of the authors and does not necessarily represent the official view of the National Cancer Institute or the National Institutes of Health. Dr M.B. Faries is a consultant for Genentech, Inc and is on the advisory board for Astellas Pharmaceuticals. Dr G.B. Deutsch and Dr D.D. Kirchoff have no relationships to disclose. Dr D.D. Kirchoff is the Harold McAlister Charitable Foundation Fellow.
Melanoma Research Program, John Wayne Cancer Institute, Providence St. John's Hospital, 2200 Santa Monica Boulevard, Santa Monica, CA 90404, USA
* Corresponding author.
E-mail address: mark.faries@jwci.org

associated with long-term survival in numerous single-institution and collaborative studies. At present, approved and investigational targeted and immunologic therapies offer improved response rates and durability of response.[4–7] Surgical therapy should play an even more important role in the management of patients with metastatic melanoma in conjunction with these expanding options of effective systemic therapies. New research will be required to determine the optimal combinations and sequences of multimodal treatment.

OPTIONS FOR SYSTEMIC THERAPY

For years, the primary modalities for treatment of metastatic melanoma consisted of single and combination cytotoxic chemotherapy regimens. Dacarbazine (DTIC) is one of the earliest and most often studied agents, approved by the US Food and Drug Administration (FDA) for treatment of advanced melanoma. Response rates for single-agent DTIC have been reported as 20% but with only 5 to 6 months' duration of response and complete response rates on the order of 5%.[8] No overall survival benefits were shown with combination chemotherapy regimens and responses remained short lived with multidrug regimens such as the Dartmouth regimen (1,3-bis (2-chloroethyl)-1-nitrosourea, DTIC, cisplatin, tamoxifen).[9]

More promising results came from the immune modulating agents, most notably interleukin-2 (IL-2). For a long time IL-2 was the only FDA-approved biologic agent approved for treatment of metastatic melanoma.[10,11] Response rates were 15% to 20% with some durable responses and significant toxicity, including pulmonary edema and shock. In a similar vein, biochemotherapy was able to increase response rates to 30% to 50%, but was never able to show improved survival (**Fig. 1**).[12–16]

Targeted and new immunologic agents have ushered in a new era of SMT. Ipilimumab (Yervoy) and vemurafenib (Zelboraf) became the first FDA-approved agents for metastatic melanoma in many years in 2011, and the first ever to show a survival benefit. Ipilimumab is a human immunoglobulin G monoclonal antibody blocking cytotoxic T lymphocyte–associated antigen 4, an immune checkpoint inhibitor. Experience with ipilimumab has yielded clinical benefit rates in 20% to 30% of stage IV patients with many durable, long-term responses.[4,17] However, immune-related adverse

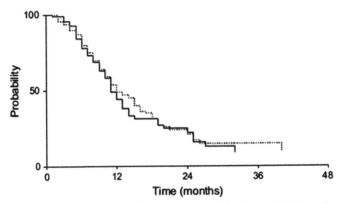

Fig. 1. Overall survival curves in the chemotherapy (*dashed*) and biochemotherapy (*solid*) arms. (*From* Bajetta E, Del Vecchio M, Nova P, et al. Multicenter phase III randomized trial of polychemotherapy (CVD regimen) versus the same chemotherapy (CT) plus subcutaneous interleukin-2 and interferon-alpha2b in metastatic melanoma. Ann Oncol 2006;17(4):575; with permission.)

events have been a well-described complication of ipilimumab and range in time of onset as well as severity. At present, vigilance and early recognition of these adverse events have led to more successful management by experienced oncologists. One of the most severe effects has been autoimmune colitis, sometimes leading to perforation and death. Management is based on the severity of the toxicity and may include cessation of ipilimumab, hydration, supportive care, symptomatic care with loperamide, budesonide, oral or intravenous steroids, and immunosuppression with infliximab.[18,19]

Vemurafenib is an inhibitor of mutated BRAF, useful for patients with the V600E mutation. The mutation is present in 40% to 60% of melanomas,[20] and, in a phase III randomized controlled trial comparing vemurafenib with dacarbazine, the almost 50% response rate was much greater than that of dacarbazine at 5% and there was an improvement in overall and progression-free survival (hazard ratio [HR], 0.37 [0.26–0.55]) in the vemurafenib arm (**Fig. 2**). Although it is useful for its rapid onset of action, BRAF inhibition remains limited by predictable brevity of response (median, 5–6 months).[5]

The latest development in the story of immune agents involves targeting of programmed cell death 1 (PD-1) and programmed cell death ligand 1 (PDL-1). Human monoclonal antibodies to PD-1 and PDL-1 are in ongoing trials with preliminary results showing improved response rates and duration of response with durable responses reported even after termination of therapy. PD-1 is a B cell–inhibitory and T cell–inhibitory receptor that binds with PDL-1 and PDL-2 to inhibit lymphocytes.[6,21,22] In a dose-escalation study of PD-1 antibody nivolumab, 107 patients with metastatic melanoma were treated between 2008 and 2012. Sixty-two percent of these patients had undergone at least 2 prior systemic treatments. Seventy-eight percent of patients had a visceral metastatic lesion and 36% had an increased lactate dehydrogenase level. Median overall survival in this population was 16.8 months with 1-year and 2-year survival rates of 62% and 43%. Objective responses were seen in 31% of all patients, and median duration of those responses was 2 years.[6]

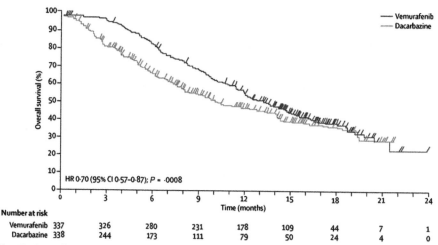

Fig. 2. Overall survival for vemurafenib (*red*) versus dacarbazine (*blue*), P = .0008. (*From* McArthur GA, Chapman PB, Robert C, et al. Safety and efficacy of vemurafenib in BRAF(V600E) and BRAF(V600K) mutation-positive melanoma (BRIM-3): extended follow-up of a phase 3, randomised, open-label study. Lancet Oncol 2014;15(3):327; with permission.)

Response rates to another PD-1 inhibitor, pembrolizumab (formerly lambrolizumab), were slightly higher at 38% across all doses in a dose-escalation study.[7] This PD-1 inhibitor is now FDA-approved as a second-line treatment of metastatic melanoma. Responses were independent of previous treatment with ipilimumab, and the adverse effects were not affected by previous exposure to ipilimumab. A study is also underway with a PDL-1 antibody, BMS-936559.[23]

Surgery in stage IV melanoma in the past has been the best option for complete response and cure for patients fortunate enough to have resectable disease. In many single-center experiences with metastasectomy for melanoma, the recurring theme is a highly selected patient population achieving favorable survival rates. Although improved responses and even immune-based cures are a reality for some patients (**Table 1**), these therapies are not the answer for all patients with advanced melanoma and surgery may play a complementary role to these therapies to achieve long-term disease control.

RATIONALE FOR SURGICAL MANAGEMENT

Although it is generally assumed that hematogenous dissemination indicates widespread metastatic disease, not amenable to local therapy, there are well-accepted examples in which metastasectomy is used as standard therapy. In colorectal cancer, for example, isolated hepatic metastases are common, and the liver may represent an end organ for tumor cells. Resection of hepatic colorectal metastases yields a clear survival benefit if the patient can be rendered free of disease, with 5-year and 10-year survival rates of 47% and 28%[24] and higher. Resection of pulmonary metastases in many cases of sarcoma is also widely accepted as a reasonable therapeutic approach.[25–27]

Metastatic melanoma may present in a wide variety of ways, varying from explosive, widespread disease to a slower-growing oligometastatic pattern. Although the mechanisms underlying these different patterns of progression are not yet known, it is evident based on the clinical behavior that in some cases the metastatic

Table 1 Selected studies involving SMT for stage IV melanoma			
Therapy (Author Name, Year)	Response Rate (Complete/Partial) (%)	Median OS (mo)	12-mo Survival % (mo)
Dacarbazine (Middleton et al,[81] 2000)	12.1 (2.7/9.4)	6.4	51 (6)
IL-2 (Atkins et al,[10] 1999)	16.0 (6.0/10.0)	11.4	—
Biochemotherapy (O'Day et al,[16] 2009)	44 (8/36)	13.5	57 (12)
Ipilimumab (Hodi et al,[4] 2010)	10.9 (1.5/9.5)	10.1	45.6 (12)
Vemurafenib (McArthur et al,[5] 2014)	57 (6/51)	13.6	39 (18)
Trametinib (Kim et al,[79] 2013)	25 (2/23)	14.2	59 (12)
Nivolumab (Topalian et al,[6] 2014)	31 (—)	16.8	62 (12)
Lambrolizumab (Hamid et al,[7] 2013)	38 (—)	—	—

Abbreviation: OS, overall survival.
Data from Refs.[4–7,10,16,79,80]

cascade is sufficiently slow to allow interruption by eradication of existing, clinically evident lesions. The oligometastatic pattern may result from intrinsic weaknesses in the tumors' ability to resist cell death, sustain proliferative signaling, evade growth suppressors, induce angiogenesis, enable replicative immortality, or activate invasion and metastasis.[28] In a situation of oligometastatic disease, that cluster of tumor cells may be the only ones with the ability to establish a metastatic deposit, and eradication of that cell population can improve outcomes or interrupt the metastatic cascade.[29]

Alternatively, the oligometastatic pattern may result from endogenous control of tumor growth or dissemination by patients' immune systems. Examples of such immune control or destruction of melanoma abound and include spontaneous regression, which is common in primary lesions and reported, although rarely, even in metastatic disease.[30] Preexisting tumor-specific antibody titers have been correlated with postmetastasectomy survival, providing evidence of the synergy of an endogenous immune response and metastasectomy. Induction of such immune protection by medical therapy, as discussed later, is another example and may lead to increased utility of metastasectomy. Surgical metastasectomy may also enhance the body's immune defenses through removal of immunosuppressive factors produced by larger metastatic lesions.[31]

Regardless of the biological mechanisms underlying long-term survival in patients after metastasectomy, resection has resulted in the highest survival rates for patients treated for stage IV melanoma, as shown in data from a large number of single-institution studies as well as larger, multicenter trials (**Table 2**).

In addition, advances in imaging, surgical techniques, and perioperative care enhance the appeal and applicability of metastasectomy. Earlier detection of metastases may be possible with the improved resolution of modern scanners and functional imaging with PET. This improved resolution could not only improve identification of patients who can undergo resection but also decrease the risk of incomplete treatment caused by missed sites of disease. Also, if improved long-term survival is the primary goal of metastasectomy, operative mortality must be reduced to the absolute minimum. However, most types of metastatic resection, even hepatic or pulmonary, can be performed with limited morbidity and extremely low mortality.[32–34]

MULTICENTER TRIALS EVALUATING METASTASECTOMY

A phase III international, randomized, placebo-controlled trial entitled Malignant Melanoma Active Immunotherapy Trial for Stage IV disease (MMAIT-IV) provides one of the largest and most complete data sets regarding outcomes of patients after metastasectomy. The study, initiated in 1998, sought to evaluate the benefit of an adjuvant melanoma vaccine (Canvaxin) plus Bacille Calmette-Guerin (BCG) compared with placebo and BCG. All patients underwent complete resection of metastatic disease before being randomized to one of the two study arms. Although the trial did not show a survival benefit associated with receiving vaccine, survival for all of the patients in the trial was greater than 40%, which was much higher than expected for patients with stage IV melanoma at the time.[35] Although it is impossible to separate the effects of selection bias or adjuvant immune stimulation with BCG from a therapeutic effect of resection, the favorable outcomes argue for strong consideration of surgery in this setting. Subsequent analysis of the trial data produced other key findings, including the prognostic significance of circulating tumor cells in the assessment of resected stage IV patients before and during adjuvant treatment.[36]

Table 2
Selected studies involving metastasectomy

| Authors/ Study | Institution | Total Patients | M1 Overall | | | | | | | | | | | |
| | | | Any Type of Surgery | | | Curative Surgery | | | Palliative/Incomplete Surgery | | | No Surgery | | |
			Patients OS	Med OS	OS at 1, 2, 3, 4, 5 y (%)	Patients OS	Med OS	OS at 1, 2, 3, 4, 5 y (%)	Patients OS	Med OS	OS at 1, 2, 3, 4, 5 y (%)	Patients OS	Med OS	OS at 1, 3, 4, 5 y (%)
Prospective Trials														
Howard et al,[33] 2012	MSLT-1	291	161	15.8	4 y = 20.8	—	—	—	—	—	—	130	6.9	4 y = 7.0
Morton et al,[35] 2006	MMAIT	496	496	32–39	5 y = 40–45	496	32–39	5 y = 40–45	—	—	—	—	—	—
Sosman et al,[37] 2011	SWOG	77	77	21.0	75/—/36/ 31/—	—	—	—	—	—	—	—	—	—
M1A														
Howard et al,[33] 2012	MSLT-1	32	26	NR	4 y = 69.3	—	—	—	—	—	—	6	12.4	4 y = 0
Essner et al,[42] 2014	JWCI	260	260	—	5 y = 25.0	—	—	—	—	—	—	—	—	—
Meyer et al,[65] 2000	Erlangen, Germany	130	—	—	—	75	17–18	5 y = 17.8–20.0	29	—	5 y = 0–16.7	26	—	5 y = 0
M1B														
Howard et al,[33] 2012	MSLT-1	49	27	17.9	4 y = 24.1	—	—	—	—	—	—	22	9.1	4 y = 14.3
Petersen et al,[44] 2007	Duke	1738	318	—	—	249	19.0	5 y = 21	69	11.0	5 y = 13	1420	6.0	5 y = 3
Neuman et al,[82] 2007	MSKCC	122	26	40.0	5 y = 29	26	40.0	5 y = 29	—	—	—	96	13.0	5 y = 0
Andrews et al,[46] 2006	Moffitt	86	86	35.0	5 y = 33	—	—	—	—	—	—	—	—	—

Study	Institution													
Essner et al,[42] 2014	JWCI	364	364	—	5 y = 21.0	—	—	—	—	—	—	—	—	—
Meyer et al,[65] 2000	Erlangen, Germany	83	130	11–14	5 y = 10.2–15.2	10	—	5 y = 50	3	—	5 y = 0	70	—	5 y = 2.3
Leo et al,[45] 2000	IRLM	328	328	17.0	5 y = 18	282	19.0	5 y = 22	46	11.0	5 y = 0	—	—	—
Ollila et al,[66] 1998	JWCI	45	45	23.1	5 y = 15.6	38	25.6	—	7	—	—	—	—	—
M1C														
Faries et al,[32] 2014 (liver)	JWCI	1078	58	24.8	5 y = 30	51	21.1	5 y = 39	7	6.2	5 y = 0	1016	8.0	5 y = 6.6
Howard et al,[33] 2012 (all)	MSLT-1	210	108	15.0	4 y = 10.5	—	—	—	—	—	—	102	6.3	4 y = 4.6
Reddy & Wolfgang,[58] 2009 (pancreas)	Johns Hopkins	11	11	14.0	5 y = 27	—	—	—	—	—	—	—	—	—
Mittendorf et al,[55] 2008 (adrenal)	MDACC	154	22	20.7	—	20	—	—	2	—	—	132	6.8	—
Collinson et al,[80] 2008 (adrenal)	Sydney	186	23	16.0	61/39/—/—/—	13	—	—	10	—	—	163	5.0	—
Fife et al,[60] 2004 (brain)	Sydney	686	205	8.7–8.9	—	—	—	—	—	—	—	446	2.1–3.4	—
Wood et al,[49] 2001 (solid organs)	JWCI	838	60	27.6	—/—/—/24	44	27.6	—/—/—/	16	8.4	5 y = 0	778	9.6	5 y = 7

(continued on next page)

Table 2
(continued)

Authors/Study	Institution	Total Patients	M1 Overall — Any Type of Surgery			Curative Surgery			Palliative/Incomplete Surgery			No Surgery		
			Patients	Med OS	OS at 1, 2, 3, 4, 5 y (%)	Patients	Med OS	OS at 1, 2, 3, 4, 5 y (%)	Patients	Med OS	OS at 1, 2, 3, 4, 5 y (%)	Patients	Med OS	OS at 1, 3, 4, 5 y (%)
Rose et al,[53] 2001 (liver)	JWCI/Sydney	923	24	28.0	—/—/41/—/29	24	28.0	—/—/41/—/29	24	28.0	—/—/41/—/29	899	6.0	5 y = 4.0
Haigh et al,[56] 1999 (adrenal)	JWCI	83	27	25.7	—	18	25.7	—	9	9.2	—	56	7.7	—
Agrawal et al,[51] 1999 (GI)	MSKCC	68	68	14.9	67/45/—/—/38	19	14.9	67/45/—/—/38	49	6.9	22/—/—/—/38	—	—	—
Ollila et al,[34] 1996 (GI)	JWCI	124	69	48.9	5 y = 41	46	48.9	5 y = 41	23	5.4	5 y = 0	55	5.7	5 y = 0

Abbreviations: GI, gastrointestinal; IRLM, International Registry of Lung Metastases; JWCI, John Wayne Cancer Institute; MDACC, MD Anderson Cancer Center; MMAIT-IV, Malignant Melanoma Active Immunotherapy Trial for Stage IV disease; MSKCC, Memorial Sloan Kettering Cancer Center; MSLT-I, Multicenter Selective Lymphadenectomy Trial; SWOG, Southwest Oncology Group.

Data from Refs. [31–33,37,42,44–46,49,51,53–56,58,60,65,66]

Another multicenter study assessing metastasectomy in patients with stage IV melanoma was the phase II randomized Southwest Oncology Group (SWOG) clinical trial (S9430). This prospective registry study enrolled subjects who were deemed completely resectable by physical examination and imaging. A total of 72 eligible subjects were enrolled, among whom 64 (89%) were found to be completely resectable at the time of surgery. Their median overall survival was 21 months, with overall survivals of 36% and 31% at 3 and 4 years, respectively (**Fig. 3**).[37] Despite its limited size, this trial confirmed that the favorable outcomes achieved through surgical resection are not limited to single institutions.

A third multicenter study that examined outcomes of patients undergoing surgical treatment of stage IV melanoma was the first Multicenter Selective Lymphadenectomy Trial (MSLT-I). Although analysis of these results was not limited to patients having complete resection, there was a high fraction of patients (55%) whose therapy on stage IV recurrence included surgery. As discussed later, the outcomes of surgically treated patients were significantly better than those of patients who received only medical treatment.

SITE-SPECIFIC SURGICAL TREATMENT
M1a Disease

American Joint Commission for Cancer melanoma staging data published in 2009 show that approximately 20% of patients with metastatic melanoma present with M1a disease (skin, soft tissue, and distant lymph nodes with normal lactate dehydrogenase), with an associated 1-year survival rate of 62%.[38] In the past, median survival varies from 10 to 24 months[39] and may be improving in the setting of increasingly effective systemic therapies. As part of a melanoma vaccine trial at the John Wayne Cancer Institute, cases of stage IV melanoma that underwent complete resection with and without adjuvant Canvaxin vaccine immunotherapy were

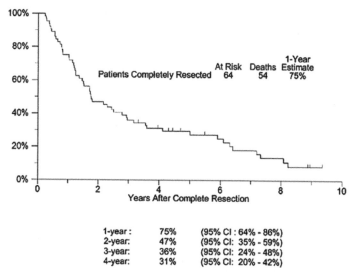

		At Risk	Deaths	1-Year Estimate
Patients Completely Resected		64	54	75%

1-year:	75%	(95% CI : 64% - 86%)
2-year:	47%	(95% CI: 35% - 59%)
3-year:	36%	(95% CI: 24% - 48%)
4-year:	31%	(95% CI: 20% - 42%)

Fig. 3. Overall survival for completely resected patients (SWOG S9430). (*From* Sosman JA, Moon J, Tuthill RJ, et al. A phase 2 trial of complete resection for stage IV melanoma: results of Southwest Oncology Group Clinical Trial S9430. Cancer 2011;117(20):4743; with permission.)

analyzed. As part of the matched-pair analysis, patients with M1a metastases who underwent metastasectomy only had a median overall survival and 5-year overall survival of 20 months and 15%, respectively, versus 41 months and 41% for those who received additional adjuvant vaccine therapy.[40] There was no statistically significant difference in overall survival in this group ($P = .13$), but outcomes overall were better than expected, potentially because of the aggressive surgical therapy that all patients received.

In MSLT-I, 32 (10%) of the 291 patients who underwent treatment of distant metastases had M1a disease. Although all patients who underwent surgery had favorable survival (vs SMT alone), those with M1a metastases did particularly well. These patients had a median survival of greater than 60 months with surgery with or without SMT versus 12.4 months with SMT alone ($P = .0106$) (**Fig. 4**A).[33] The highly selected population of patients in MSLT-I, many of whom received medical therapy, had a significantly higher survival with surgical treatment than any previously reported experience. These outcomes are superior to those of many patients with stage III metastases.

Within the M1a cohort, patients with skin and soft tissue metastases have better outcomes with surgery than those with distant lymph node disease. Often these patients can become symptomatic from their disease, necessitating palliative resection to control pain, ulceration, or bleeding. Technical considerations in metastasectomy in these patients have not been thoroughly studied. However, because complete resection seems desirable based on prior survival comparisons with incomplete resection, negative resection margins are desirable. In the setting of lymph node metastases, complete dissection of the involved basin has been recommended, although high-quality data addressing the necessary extent of node dissection in this setting are lacking.[41]

M1b Disease

The pulmonary system is the most common site of metastatic disease in melanoma, comprising approximately 40% of all M1 disease.[42] At 1 year from diagnosis of metastatic melanoma, survival for M1b patients (lung metastases) is 53%, which is superior to survival for M1c disease (other visceral metastases).[38] However, by 2 years the survival advantage disappears and prognosis remains similar thereafter.[43] In a post-hoc analysis of MSLT-I data, M1b patients treated surgically with or without SMT had a median survival of 17.9 months versus 9.1 months for medical treatment alone ($P = .1143$) (see **Fig. 4**B).[33] Although this difference is not statistically significant, the trend is consistent with prior data regarding favorable survival among surgically treated patients. Patient selection is paramount in order to identify patients most likely to benefit from surgery.

Multiple retrospective reports examined the surgical treatment of melanoma lung metastases.[44] Leo and colleagues[45] in 2000 tried to define the ideal population to benefit from metastasectomy by using 3 significant factors: time to development of pulmonary metastases, number of pulmonary metastases, and completeness of metastasectomy. Patients with complete metastasectomy, long disease-free interval (>36 months), and an isolated metastasis (group I) had the best outcome, with 5-year and 10-year survivals of 29% and 26%, respectively. Patients who had a complete metastasectomy with either multiple metastases or short pulmonary metastasis–free survival (group II) had a 20% and 11% survival at 5 and 10 years, respectively. Patients who had a short time to development of lung metastases and multiple lesions (group III) or an incomplete metastasectomy (group IV) did the poorest, with only 7% surviving 5 years in group III and no survivors in group IV. Other experiences with isolated

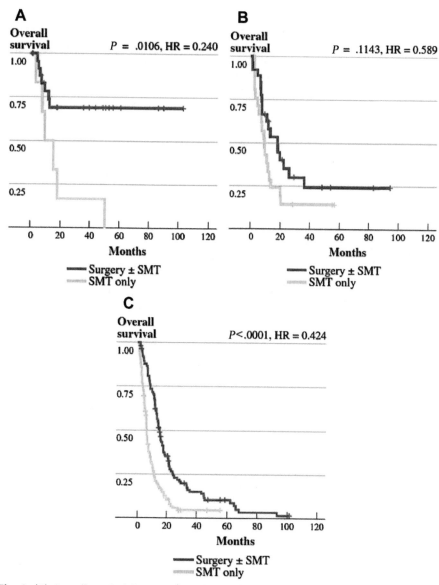

Fig. 4. (*A*) Overall survival for patients with M1a recurrence treated with surgery with or without SMT versus SMT alone. (*B*) Overall survival for patients with M1b recurrence treated with surgery with or without SMT versus SMT alone. (*C*) Overall survival for patients with M1c recurrence treated with surgery with or without SMT versus SMT alone. (*From* Howard JH, Thompson JF, Mozzillo N, et al. Metastasectomy for distant metastatic melanoma: analysis of data from the first Multicenter Selective Lymphadenectomy Trial (MSLT-I). Ann Surg Oncol 2012;19:2551; with permission.)

pulmonary metastasectomy have reported similar results with 33% of patients surviving 5 years.[46]

Pulmonary metastases are generally asymptomatic and discovered incidentally on imaging performed for surveillance or staging purposes. Often patients with melanoma have benign pulmonary findings on imaging, which may be misinterpreted as metastatic disease. The value of baseline imaging cannot be understated, particularly in evaluating the lungs. Using serial imaging to closely evaluate pulmonary metastases for interval growth can be valuable in surgical decision making.

Technical considerations for pulmonary metastasectomy include consideration of concomitant nodal staging. Lymphatic mapping from pulmonary metastases has been reported and seems technically feasible, but is challenging. The pathologic status of these sentinel nodes for the metastatic site seem to carry significant prognostic information.[47] In addition, it seems that even modern radiographic imaging may not be adequate to identify all pulmonary metastases preoperatively. Because complete resection seems preferable, this argues for the continued use of open surgical procedures that enable palpation of the lung rather than thoracoscopic approaches.[48]

M1c Disease

Patients with M1c disease can also present silently, as an incidental finding on imaging studies. However, depending on the location, these tumors can be symptomatic. Gastrointestinal (GI) metastases can result in clinically apparent bleeding, but more frequently are occult, presenting as anemia. Other solid organs (liver, spleen, and so forth) can be associated with pain secondary to stretching of the capsule. Rupture and associated hemorrhage are rare, but can be catastrophic. The resection of intra-abdominal melanoma metastases has been associated with an improved survival, independent of the number of metastatic sites.[49] In MSLT-I, M1c patients who underwent surgery with or without accompanying medical therapy had a 15.0-month median survival compared with 6.3 months for those treated with SMT alone (P<.0001) (see **Fig. 4C**).[33]

Several studies have focused on specific organ systems and outcomes after directed metastasectomy. Approximately 50% of patients with metastatic melanoma have GI metastases in autopsy series.[50] The most common site of single-organ involvement was the small intestine, seen in about 70% of patients with GI disease. The colon, stomach, and rectum, in order of occurrence, account for the rest of the involved GI sites. Ollila and colleagues[34] reported a series of 124 patients with GI metastases, 69 of whom underwent surgical resection (66% with curative intent). Median survival was 48.9 months in the curative surgical group versus 5.4 months and 5.7 months in the palliative resection and medical therapy groups, respectively (P<.001). Patients who underwent complete resection with the GI tract as the first site of distant disease had superior survival outcomes. Agrawal and colleagues[51] determined that, in addition to complete metastasectomy, low preoperative serum lactate dehydrogenase was also an independent favorable prognostic factor. Although palliative resection is not associated with long-term survival, it often successfully alleviates symptoms of pain, bleeding, or obstruction.

Hepatic resection or ablation of melanoma metastases have been reported in the literature.[52–54] A recent article by Faries and colleagues[32] reevaluated the role of surgical resection in hepatic melanoma metastases in the current era of effective systemic therapy. Median and 5-year overall survival was 24.8 months and 30%, respectively, for surgical patients versus 8 months and 6.6%, respectively, for those treated medically (P<.001). The type of surgical therapy (ablation, resection, and so forth) did not differentially affect outcomes. Completeness of metastasectomy and stabilization of melanoma on therapy before surgical resection predicted an improved overall survival. Patients with any benefit from systemic treatment (response or disease stabilization) may particularly benefit from surgical consolidation.

Adrenal metastasectomy is not common, but several cases have been reported in the literature. The largest report of adrenal metastases from melanoma included 154 patients, 22 of whom underwent adrenalectomy. The median overall survival for resected patients was 20.7 months, compared with 6.8 months for those managed nonoperatively (P<.0001).[55] In a similar cohort from the John Wayne Cancer Institute, median survival was 25.7 months for patients who underwent complete resection.[56] Cases with synchronous, unresectable disease fared much worse than those with isolated adrenal metastases, reiterating the importance of patient selection. Isolated pancreatic melanoma metastases are exceedingly rare, but can also be successfully treated with surgical resection in highly selected cases.[57] One of the largest experiences, by Reddy and Wolfgang,[58] reported a median and 5-year survival of 14 months and 27%, respectively, in pancreatic melanoma metastases (n = 11) treated surgically. The median time to metastasectomy was 4 years from excision of the primary melanoma.

Brain metastases occur in at least 15% to 40% of patients with stage IV melanoma, with an even higher incidence reported in autopsy studies. The M1 stage (M1b or M1c) and lactate dehydrogenase level at diagnosis of unresectable stage III/IV can predict the risk for the development of brain metastases.[59] At present, almost all patients who undergo craniotomy receive adjuvant radiotherapy in the form of stereotactic radiosurgery or whole-brain radiation. In one of the largest studies reported to date, patients treated with surgery and postoperative radiotherapy (n = 158) had a median survival of 8.9 months versus 8.7 months and 3.4 months for surgery alone (n = 47) and radiotherapy alone (n = 236), respectively. Patients receiving supportive care (n = 210) had a median survival of 2.1 months.[60] Lonser and colleagues[61] analyzed consecutive patients with brain metastases treated with immunotherapy (IL-2 and vaccine in most) and surgery at the National Institutes of Health. They found an improved outcome in patients showing objective response to immunotherapy (median survival of 34 months vs 17 months; P = .02). Rate of local control was 92.5% overall, and postoperative whole-brain radiation therapy did not seem to affect local recurrence. In metastatic melanoma with brain metastases, metastasectomy is indicated in most patients, whether palliative or curative. Patients with isolated cerebral metastases, absent or stable extracranial disease, and no preoperative neurologic deficits may derive the greatest benefit.[62–64]

Factors That Affect the Decision to Perform Metastasectomy

Appropriate selection of patients for metastasectomy can be challenging, but is critically important. Avoiding operation in patients who are likely to have an early postoperative disease recurrence is desirable, as is selecting patients likely to achieve long-term survival. Although no high-level data are available to provide true predictive measures, several factors seem to be of value, based on reported series.

COMPLETE RESECTABILITY VERSUS CYTOREDUCTION

One factor that has been consistently shown to be required for extended postoperative survival is the completeness of resection. Complete metastasectomy, rendering the patient with no evidence of disease, results in far superior outcomes compared with cytoreductive or palliative surgery. Meyer and colleagues[65] showed that surgical therapy for distant metastases was most beneficial when all disease could be removed (**Fig. 5**). Median survival rates for curative versus incomplete resection were 17 months and 6 months, respectively. Carefully choosing this population depends on advanced imaging technology and surgical judgment and experience. Based on the SWOG registry study, it seems that complete resectability can be accurately predicted in about 9 out of 10 cases.[37] As in all surgical decisions, balancing the

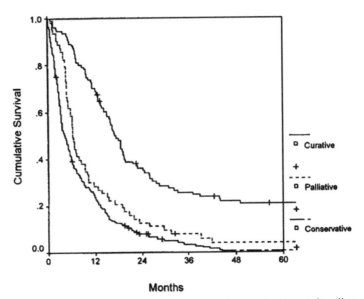

Fig. 5. Cumulative survival for stage IV patients according to treatment (top line, curative; middle line, palliative; bottom line, conservative). (*From* Meyer T, Merkel S, Goehl J, et al. Surgical therapy for distant metastases of malignant melanoma. Cancer 2000;89:1989; with permission.)

morbidity and mortality from a planned metastasectomy with its potential benefit is critical. Patients with good preoperative performance status may be most likely to have a rapid postoperative recovery. In the era of increasingly effective systemic therapies, such a rapid return of function is clearly desirable.

TUMOR DOUBLING TIME AND DISEASE-FREE INTERVAL

There is broad agreement that patients with indolent, oligometastatic melanoma are optimal candidates for resection, whereas those with rapidly progressive disease are not. However, no currently available test allows a precise measurement of the biological aggressiveness of metastatic disease. Some indirect means of assessment are available, including disease-free interval and tumor volume doubling time (TVDT). A longer disease-free interval suggests slow metastatic progression, which should lead to more favorable postresection survival. A disease-free interval of greater than 36 months from melanoma diagnosis to the occurrence of metastatic disease is associated with an improved overall survival. Although patients generally present with only 1 initial imaging study to provide a measure of the size of their metastases, serial imaging often occurs over the course of a work-up of that disease, or is typically available as patients undergo SMT. These serial measurements allow an assessment of the speed of growth of a tumor, measured as TVDT. Ollila and colleagues,[66] in pulmonary melanoma metastases, showed that a TVDT of at least 60 days is prognostic, with an associated median survival of 29.2 months, versus 23.1 months for a TVDT less than 60 months ($P<.0001$).

RESPONSE TO SYSTEMIC MEDICAL THERAPY

In several other cancer types, response to medical therapy has been determined to be a powerful selection tool for metastasectomy. This finding is well shown by the dominant effect response to chemotherapy has on the prognosis of patients undergoing resection of hepatic colorectal metastases.[67] In melanoma, the lack of efficacy of systemic treatments in the past has limited the ability to use this factor in patient selection. However, with current drugs, the potential for surgical consolidation of an initial medical response is an increasingly attractive and likely scenario. A recently reported series of hepatic surgery for metastatic melanoma showed substantially improved outcomes among patients who had either response or stabilization of disease before resection.[32]

There is some evidence that patients who experience complete surgical remission after medical treatment have comparable survival outcomes with those who have a complete response to SMT.[68] In the setting of IL-2–based immunotherapy, salvage surgery among patients with partial response or recurrence after complete response can achieve cure in 20% of patients and survival greater than 5 years in 36% of patients.[69] This paradigm has been described in several other cancers, including GI, breast, and sarcoma, with liver, lung, and adrenal metastases.[70–72]

PALLIATION

Specific metastatic lesions may lead to symptoms that are amenable to surgical treatment. These lesions include the GI tract, where metastases may lead to obstruction, bleeding, or pain. Superficial skin or soft tissue lesions may also bleed or cause pain and may lead to difficulties with necrosis and superinfection. Brain metastases may be symptomatic even when small, often because of surrounding vasogenic edema. These symptoms may not only decrease the patients' quality of life but also limit their ability to undergo systemic therapy. Resection of these problematic lesions remains a consideration for these reasons, even when complete resection of all metastatic sites is not possible. Symptomatic relief is most often achieved with the surgical resection of lung and abdominal metastases but also in most patients with skin, soft tissue, and brain metastases.[73] The balance of the morbidity of a palliative resection and the quality-of-life benefits that may be obtained is clear in some cases, but can be challenging clinical judgments in others.

FUTURE INTERSECTIONS OF SYSTEMIC THERAPY AND SURGERY

For many years, resection was the only therapy for stage IV disease associated with substantial rates of long-term survival. With the development of modern, more effective drug therapies, the situation has become more complex. One challenge this has created is in determining the optimal combination and sequence of therapies for each patient. As noted earlier, patients who first undergo partially effective drug therapy seem to have particularly favorable outcomes after surgical consolidation. However, which resectable patients should first have a period of medical treatment is unknown.

Alternatively, patients who receive a medical treatment that is initially effective but who then develop limited sites of disease progression may benefit from selective resection of those problematic lesions, while continuing on the otherwise effective drug. This surgical sniping may extend the period of disease control and postpone the need to change therapies. Preliminary support for this idea can be seen in the setting of resistance to BRAF inhibition.[74] Furthermore, clinicians are using approved SMT in the neoadjuvant setting for locally advanced melanoma, as well as those with metastatic disease. Several early reports and case studies have yielded promising results.[75–78]

Surgery is also a component of some adoptive immunotherapy strategies in which tumor is resected and the responsive immune cells within the lesion are isolated and amplified to produce a cell product that can be returned to the patient. This strategy has been successfully used, initially at the National Cancer Institute, and now at several other centers around the world.[69,70]

Overall, this new, complex situation, although confusing, is an important opportunity for continued progress in the treatment of metastatic melanoma. A great deal of research will be required to determine optimal treatment algorithms, but it seems that surgery should continue to play a prominent role.

REFERENCES

1. Siegel R, Naishadham D, Jemal A. Cancer statistics, 2013. CA Cancer J Clin 2013;63:11–30.
2. Barth A, Wanek LA, Morton DL. Prognostic factors in 1,521 melanoma patients with distant metastases. J Am Coll Surg 1995;181(3):193–201.
3. Korn EL, Liu PY, Lee SJ, et al. Meta-analysis of phase II cooperative group trials in metastatic stage IV melanoma to determine progression-free and overall survival benchmarks for future phase II trials. J Clin Oncol 2008;26(4): 527–34.
4. Hodi FS, O'Day SJ, McDermott DF, et al. Improved survival with ipilimumab in patients with metastatic melanoma. N Engl J Med 2010;363(8):711–23.
5. McArthur GA, Chapman PB, Robert C, et al. Safety and efficacy of vemurafenib in BRAF(V600E) and BRAF(V600K) mutation-positive melanoma (BRIM-3): extended follow-up of a phase 3, randomised, open-label study. Lancet Oncol 2014;15(3):323–32.
6. Topalian SL, Sznol M, McDermott DF, et al. Survival, durable tumor remission, and long-term safety in patients with advanced melanoma receiving nivolumab. J Clin Oncol 2014;32(10):1020–30.
7. Hamid O, Robert C, Daud A, et al. Safety and tumor responses with lambrolizumab (anti-PD-1) in melanoma. N Engl J Med 2013;369(2):134–44.
8. Serrone L, Zeuli M, Sega FM, et al. Dacarbazine-based chemotherapy for metastatic melanoma: thirty-year experience overview. J Exp Clin Cancer Res 2000; 19(1):21–34.
9. Del Prete SA, Maurer LH, O'Donnell J, et al. Combination chemotherapy with cisplatin, carmustine, dacarbazine, and tamoxifen in metastatic melanoma. Cancer Treat Rep 1984;68(11):1403–5.
10. Atkins MB, Lotze MT, Dutcher JP, et al. High-dose recombinant interleukin 2 therapy for patients with metastatic melanoma: analysis of 270 patients treated between 1985 and 1993. J Clin Oncol 1999;17(7):2105–16.
11. Rosenberg SA, Yang JC, Topalian SL, et al. Treatment of 283 consecutive patients with metastatic melanoma or renal cell cancer using high-dose bolus interleukin 2. JAMA 1994;271(12):907–13.
12. O'Day SJ, Gammon G, Boasberg PD, et al. Advantages of concurrent biochemotherapy modified by decrescendo interleukin-2, granulocyte colony-stimulating factor, and tamoxifen for patients with metastatic melanoma. J Clin Oncol 1999;17(9):2752–61.
13. Bajetta E, Del Vecchio M, Nova P, et al. Multicenter phase III randomized trial of polychemotherapy (CVD regimen) versus the same chemotherapy (CT) plus subcutaneous interleukin-2 and interferon-alpha2b in metastatic melanoma. Ann Oncol 2006;17(4):571–7.
14. Rosenberg SA, Yang JC, Schwartzentruber DJ, et al. Prospective randomized trial of the treatment of patients with metastatic melanoma using chemotherapy

with cisplatin, dacarbazine, and tamoxifen alone or in combination with interleukin-2 and interferon alfa-2b. J Clin Oncol 1999;17(3):968–75.

15. Eton O, Legha SS, Bedikian AY, et al. Sequential biochemotherapy versus chemotherapy for metastatic melanoma: results from a phase III randomized trial. J Clin Oncol 2002;20(8):2045–52.

16. O'Day SJ, Atkins MB, Boasberg P, et al. Phase II multicenter trial of maintenance biotherapy after induction concurrent biochemotherapy for patients with metastatic melanoma. J Clin Oncol 2009;27(36):6207–12.

17. Wolchok JD, Weber JS, Maio M, et al. Four-year survival rates for patients with metastatic melanoma who received ipilimumab in phase II clinical trials. Ann Oncol 2013;24(8):2174–80.

18. Weber JS, Dummer R, de Pril V, et al. Patterns of onset and resolution of immune-related adverse events of special interest with ipilimumab: detailed safety analysis from a phase 3 trial in patients with advanced melanoma. Cancer 2013; 119(9):1675–82.

19. Fecher LA, Agarwala SS, Hodi FS, et al. Ipilimumab and its toxicities: a multidisciplinary approach. Oncologist 2013;18(6):733–43.

20. Davies H, Bignell GR, Cox C, et al. Mutations of the BRAF gene in human cancer. Nature 2002;417(6892):949–54.

21. Dong H, Strome SE, Salomao DR, et al. Tumor-associated B7-H1 promotes T-cell apoptosis: a potential mechanism of immune evasion. Nat Med 2002;8(8): 793–800.

22. Topalian SL, Hodi FS, Brahmer JR, et al. Safety, activity, and immune correlates of anti-PD-1 antibody in cancer. N Engl J Med 2012;366(26):2443–54.

23. Brahmer JR, Tykodi SS, Chow LQ, et al. Safety and activity of anti-PD-L1 antibody in patients with advanced cancer. N Engl J Med 2012;366(26): 2455–65.

24. Wei AC, Greig PD, Grant D, et al. Survival after hepatic resection for colorectal metastases: a 10-year experience. Ann Surg Oncol 2006;13(5):668–76.

25. Abdalla EK, Pisters PW. Metastasectomy for limited metastases from soft tissue sarcoma. Curr Treat Options Oncol 2002;3(6):497–505.

26. Winkler K, Torggler S, Beron G, et al. Results of treatment in primary disseminated osteosarcoma. Analysis of the follow-up of patients in the cooperative osteosarcoma studies COSS-80 and COSS-82. Onkologie 1989;12(2):92–6 [in German].

27. Bacci G, Mercuri M, Briccoli A, et al. Osteogenic sarcoma of the extremity with detectable lung metastases at presentation. Results of treatment of 23 patients with chemotherapy followed by simultaneous resection of primary and metastatic lesions. Cancer 1997;79(2):245–54.

28. Hanahan D, Weinberg RA. Hallmarks of cancer: The next generation. Cell 2011; 144(5):646–74.

29. Roth JA, Silverstein MJ, Morton DL. Metastatic potential of metastases. Surgery 1976;79(6):669–73.

30. Bramhall RJ, Mahady K, Peach AH. Spontaneous regression of metastatic melanoma - clinical evidence of the abscopal effect. Eur J Surg Oncol 2014;40(1): 34–41.

31. Hsueh EC, Gupta RK, Yee R, et al. Does endogenous immune response determine the outcome of surgical therapy for metastatic melanoma? Ann Surg Oncol 2000;7(3):232–8.

32. Faries MB, Leung A, Morton DL, et al. A 20-year experience of hepatic resection for melanoma: is there an expanding role? J Am Coll Surg 2014;219(1):62–8.

33. Howard JH, Thompson JF, Mozzillo N, et al. Metastasectomy for distant metastatic melanoma: analysis of data from the first Multicenter Selective Lymphadenectomy Trial (MSLT-I). Ann Surg Oncol 2012;19(8):2547–55.

34. Ollila DW, Essner R, Wanek LA, et al. Surgical resection for melanoma metastatic to the gastrointestinal tract. Arch Surg 1996;131(9):975–9, 979–80.

35. Morton DL, Mozzillo N, Thompson JA, et al. Multicenter double-blind phase III trial of Canvaxin vs. placebo as post-surgical adjuvant in metastatic melanoma. In: Society of Surgical Oncology 59th Annual Cancer Symposium, March 23–26. San Diego (CA), 2006.

36. Hoshimoto S, Faries MB, Morton DL, et al. Assessment of prognostic circulating tumor cells in a phase III trial of adjuvant immunotherapy after complete resection of stage IV melanoma. Ann Surg 2012;255(2):357–62.

37. Sosman JA, Moon J, Tuthill RJ, et al. A phase 2 trial of complete resection for stage IV melanoma: results of Southwest Oncology Group Clinical Trial S9430. Cancer 2011;117(20):4740–6.

38. Balch CM, Gershenwald JE, Soong SJ, et al. Final version of 2009 AJCC melanoma staging and classification. J Clin Oncol 2009;27:6199–206.

39. Ollila DW. Complete metastasectomy in patients with stage IV metastatic melanoma. Lancet Oncol 2006;7(11):919–24.

40. Hsueh EC, Essner R, Foshag LJ, et al. Prolonged survival after complete resection of disseminated melanoma and active immunotherapy with a therapeutic cancer vaccine. J Clin Oncol 2002;20(23):4549–54.

41. Martinez SR, Young SE. A rational surgical approach to the treatment of distant melanoma metastases. Cancer Treat Rev 2008;34:614–20.

42. Essner R, Lee JH, Wanek LA, et al. Contemporary surgical treatment of advanced-stage melanoma. Arch Surg 2004;139:961–6 [discussion: 966–7].

43. Balch CM, Soong SJ, Gershenwald JE, et al. Prognostic factors analysis of 17,600 melanoma patients: validation of the American Joint Committee on Cancer melanoma staging system. J Clin Oncol 2001;19:3622–34.

44. Petersen RP, Hanish SI, Haney JC, et al. Improved survival with pulmonary metastasectomy: an analysis of 1720 patients with pulmonary metastatic melanoma. J Thorac Cardiovasc Surg 2007;133(1):104–10.

45. Leo F, Cagini L, Rocmans P, et al. Lung metastases from melanoma: when is surgical treatment warranted? Br J Cancer 2000;83:569–72.

46. Andrews S, Robinson L, Cantor A, et al. Survival after surgical resection of isolated pulmonary metastases from malignant melanoma. Cancer Control 2006; 13:218–23.

47. Faries MB, Bleicher RJ, Ye X, et al. Lymphatic mapping and sentinel lymphadenectomy for primary and metastatic pulmonary malignant neoplasms. Arch Surg 2004;139(8):870–6 [discussion: 876–7].

48. Kidner TB, Yoon J, Faries MB, et al. Preoperative imaging of pulmonary metastases in patients with melanoma: implications for minimally invasive techniques. Arch Surg 2012;147(9):871–4.

49. Wood TF, DiFronzo LA, Rose DM, et al. Does complete resection of melanoma metastatic to solid intra-abdominal organs improve survival? Ann Surg Oncol 2001;8(8):658–62.

50. Ollila DW, Gleisner AL, Hsueh EC. Rationale for complete metastasectomy in patients with stage IV metastatic melanoma. J Surg Oncol 2011;104:420–4.

51. Agrawal S, Yao TJ, Coit DG. Surgery for melanoma metastatic to the gastrointestinal tract. Ann Surg Oncol 1999;6(4):336–44.

52. Pawlik TM, Zorzi D, Abdalla EK, et al. Hepatic resection for metastatic melanoma: distinct patterns of recurrence and prognosis for ocular versus cutaneous disease. Ann Surg Oncol 2006;13:712–20.

53. Rose DM, Essner R, Hughes TM, et al. Surgical resection for metastatic melanoma to the liver: the John Wayne Cancer Institute and Sydney Melanoma Unit experience. Arch Surg 2001;136:950–5.

54. Mariani P, Piperno-Neumann S, Servois V, et al. Surgical management of liver metastases from uveal melanoma: 16 years' experience at the Institut Curie. Eur J Surg Oncol 2009;35:1192–7.

55. Mittendorf EA, Lim SJ, Schacherer CW, et al. Melanoma adrenal metastasis: natural history and surgical management. Am J Surg 2008;195(3):363–8 [discussion: 368–9].

56. Haigh PI, Essner R, Wardlaw JC, et al. Long-term survival after complete resection of melanoma metastatic to the adrenal gland. Ann Surg Oncol 1999;6(7): 633–9.

57. Goyal J, Lipson EJ, Rezaee N, et al. Surgical resection of malignant melanoma metastatic to the pancreas: case series and review of literature. J Gastrointest Cancer 2012;43(3):431–6.

58. Reddy S, Wolfgang CL. The role of surgery in the management of isolated metastases to the pancreas. Lancet Oncol 2009;10(3):287–93.

59. Bedikian AY, Wei C, Detry M, et al. Predictive factors for the development of brain metastasis in advanced unresectable metastatic melanoma. Am J Clin Oncol 2011;34:603–10.

60. Fife KM, Colman MH, Stevens GN, et al. Determinants of outcome in melanoma patients with cerebral metastases. J Clin Oncol 2004;22:1293–300.

61. Lonser RR, Song DK, Klapper J, et al. Surgical management of melanoma brain metastases in patients treated with immunotherapy. J Neurosurg 2011;115(1):30–6.

62. Wroński M, Arbit E. Surgical treatment of brain metastases from melanoma: a retrospective study of 91 patients. J Neurosurg 2000;93:9–18.

63. Konstadoulakis MM, Messaris E, Zografos G, et al. Prognostic factors in malignant melanoma patients with solitary or multiple brain metastases. Is there a role for surgery? J Neurosurg Sci 2000;44:211–8 [discussion: 219].

64. Sampson JH, Carter JH, Friedman AH, et al. Demographics, prognosis, and therapy in 702 patients with brain metastases from malignant melanoma. J Neurosurg 1998;88:11–20.

65. Meyer T, Merkel S, Goehl J, et al. Surgical therapy for distant metastases of malignant melanoma. Cancer 2000;89:1983–91.

66. Ollila DW, Stern SL, Morton DL. Tumor doubling time: a selection factor for pulmonary resection of metastatic melanoma. J Surg Oncol 1998;69:206–11.

67. Brouquet A, Abdalla EK, Kopetz S, et al. High survival rate after two-stage resection of advanced colorectal liver metastases: response-based selection and complete resection define outcome. J Clin Oncol 2011;29(8):1083–90.

68. O'Day S, Boasberg P. Management of metastatic melanoma 2005. Surg Oncol Clin North Am 2006;15:419–37.

69. Yang JC, Abad J, Sherry R. Treatment of oligometastases after successful immunotherapy. Semin Radiat Oncol 2006;16:131–5.

70. Weichselbaum RR, Hellman S. Oligometastases revisited. Nat Rev Clin Oncol 2011;8:378–82.

71. Niibe Y, Hayakawa K. Oligometastases and oligo-recurrence: the new era of cancer therapy. Jpn J Clin Oncol 2010;40:107–11.

72. Lo SS, Moffatt-Bruce SD, Dawson LA, et al. The role of local therapy in the management of lung and liver oligometastases. Nat Rev Clin Oncol 2011;8:405–16.

73. Wornom IL, Smith JW, Soong SJ, et al. Surgery as palliative treatment for distant metastases of melanoma. Ann Surg 1986;204(2):181–5.

74. Kim KB. Pattern and outcome of disease progression in phase I study of vemurafenib in patients with metastatic melanoma. ASCO Annual Meeting, June 3–7. Chicago (IL), 2011.

75. Laks S, Brueske KA, Hsueh EC. Neoadjuvant treatment of melanoma: case reports and review. Exp Hematol Oncol 2013;2:30.

76. Kolar GR, Miller-Thomas MM, Schmidt RE, et al. Neoadjuvant treatment of a solitary melanoma brain metastasis with vemurafenib. J Clin Oncol 2013;31(3): e40–3.

77. Tarhini AA, Edington H, Butterfield LH, et al. Immune monitoring of the circulation and the tumor microenvironment in patients with regionally advanced melanoma receiving neoadjuvant ipilimumab. PLoS One 2014;9(2):e87705.

78. La Greca M, Grasso G, Antonelli G, et al. Neoadjuvant therapy for locally advanced melanoma: new strategies with targeted therapies. Onco Targets Ther 2014;7:1115–21.

79. Kim KB, Kefford R, Pavlick AC, et al. Phase II study of the MEK1/MEK2 inhibitor trametinib in patients with metastatic *BRAF*-mutant cutaneous melanoma previously treated with or without a BRAF inhibitor. J Clin Oncol 2013;31(4):482–9.

80. Collinson FJ, Lam TK, Bruijn WM, et al. Long-term survival and occasional regression of distant melanoma metastases after adrenal metastasectomy. Ann Surg Oncol 2008;15(6):1741–9.

81. Middleton MR, Grob JJ, Aaronson N, et al. Randomized phase III study of temozolomide versus dacarbazine in the treatment of patients with metastatic malignant melanoma. J Clin Oncol 2000;18(1):158–66.

82. Neuman HB, Patel A, Hanlon C, et al. Stage IV melanoma and pulmonary metastases: factors predictive of survival. Ann Surg Oncol 2007;14(10):2847–53.

Intralesional Therapy for In-transit and Satellite Metastases in Melanoma

Kendra J. Feeney, MD*, Michael J. Mastrangelo, MD

KEYWORDS

- Intralesional therapy • Bacille Calmette-Guerin • Vaccinia • Scarification
- Granulocyte-macrophage colony-stimulating factor • Rose bengal • Melanoma
- In-transit disease

KEY POINTS

- Agents such as bacille Calmette-Guerin, interleukin-2, interferon, rose bengal, and granulocyte-macrophage colony-stimulating factor/viral recombinants are viable options for treatment of local-regional dermal and subcutaneous melanoma metastases through intralesional injections.
- Remission rates are significantly higher than when they are used systemically to treat metastatic disease, suggesting that the concentration of the agent within the tumor is a significant factor in determining response.
- The mechanism of the antitumor effect is postulated to be immunologic but a bystander effect caused by the inflammatory response is also possible.

INTRODUCTION

Intratumoral therapy with bacteria/bacterial products dates to at least the 1890s.[1] It was in 1893 that William Coley published his case series of the deliberate infection of sarcomas with a mixture of *Streptococcus pyogenes* and *Serratia marcescens*. He concluded that bacterial infection could induce tumor regression. A scientific basis for this claim was provided by Zbar and Rapp[2] who showed regression of subcutaneous implants of a diethyl-nitrosamine–induced hepatocellular carcinoma in inbred strain-2 male guinea pigs by intratumor injection of bacille Calmette-Guerin (BCG) with regression not only of the injected tumor but also regression of regional nodal

Disclosures: The authors have nothing to disclose.
Department of Medical Oncology, Sidney Kimmel School of Medicine, Thomas Jefferson University, 1025 Walnut Street, Suite 700, Philadelphia, PA 19107, USA
* Corresponding author. Department of Medical Oncology, 1025 Walnut Street, Suite 700, Philadelphia, PA 19107.
E-mail address: kendra.feeney@jefferson.edu

Surg Oncol Clin N Am 24 (2015) 299–308
http://dx.doi.org/10.1016/j.soc.2014.12.007
1055-3207/15/$ – see front matter © 2015 Elsevier Inc. All rights reserved.

surgonc.theclinics.com

metastases. The animals were resistant to rechallenge with the same tumor.[2] This finding sparked renewed interest in intratumoral therapy as an approach not only to local tumor regression but also to inducing systemic antitumor immunity.

Over the ensuing decades, intratumoral therapy has expanded beyond the use of microbes and microbial products (eg, BCG, methanol extraction residue of BCG, purified protein derivative of *Mycobacterium tuberculosis*, vaccinia, *Clostridium novyi* NT [no toxin]) to chemicals (eg, dinitrochlorobenzene, rose bengal), cancer chemotherapeutic agents (eg, nitrogen mustard, 5-fluorouracil, imiquimod), cytokines (eg, interferon, interleukin-2 [IL-2], granulocyte-macrophage colony-stimulating factor [GM-CSF]), recombinant organisms (eg, vaccinia/GM-CSF, herpes simplex/GM-CSF, fowlpox/tumor antigen), and hybrid molecules (eg, mesothelin-diphtheria toxin gene). This list is incomplete and is being added to on a regular basis.

The obvious appeal of the intratumoral (intralesional/topical) approach to therapy is the ability to deliver a high concentration of the therapeutic agent directly to the tumor, usually with minimal systemic effects. The clinical experience in melanoma with the most extensively studied agents is reviewed in this article. Although regression of systemic disease has been more elusive, locoregional response rates approach 90%. We have found this approach invaluable in the treatment of dermal satellite and in-transit metastases, particularly those in cosmetically or functionally eloquent areas and also when the lesions encompass a large area defying surgical excision. This treatment can also be applicable in frail or medically compromised patients. To encourage more widespread application, this article provides detailed instructions on the use of some commercially available agents, such as BCG and the cytokines.

VACCINIA

Vaccinia is a large poxvirus with a double-stranded DNA genome that closely resembles cowpox. It is the active constituent of the vaccine that eradicated smallpox. Vaccination has been discontinued and thus a large segment of the population is unprotected. Because of bioterrorism concerns, the vaccine is sequestered and no longer available for clinical use. Use in cancer treatment was prompted by its oncolytic nature and the ability of the virus to activate macrophages, professional antigen-presenting cells. This ability in turn could enhance systemic immunity. Vaccinia virus has been used for intralesional therapy for cutaneous melanoma.

In 1961, Belisario and Milton[3] reported treating a 29-year-old woman with extensive in-transit deposits of melanoma with vaccinia virus intralesionally. All injected lesions resolved or decreased in size. Their work continued into the 1970s, studying both intralesional vaccinia and systemic immunization. Everall and colleagues[4] reported a series of 48 patients with primary melanomas who were randomized to having the primary lesion injected with vaccinia 2 weeks before excision versus primary excision alone. Relapse-free survival was improved in the patients treated with vaccinia.

In anticipation of using vaccinia as a vector, Mastrangelo and colleagues[5] treated 5 patients with metastatic melanoma accessible to injection with intralesional therapy with the wild-type vaccinia. All patients developed antivaccinia antibody titers. Despite this, infectivity could be maintained with repeat treatments. The injections were well tolerated. There were 1 complete (10+ years' duration) and 3 partial remissions. However, this product is no longer available.

BACILLE CALMETTE-GUERIN

BCG is prepared from an attenuated strain of *Mycobacterium bovis*. It is similar enough to its wild ancestors to provide immunity against *M tuberculosis* (its original application was in the prevention of tuberculosis). BCG induces an intense inflammatory response at injection sites, triggering cytokine cascade and macrophage activation. Direct tumor cell killing is a bystander effect of the inflammation and systemic effects are mediated via its ability to activate macrophages, professional antigen-presenting cells. The ability of BCG to induce an antitumor immune response was shown by Zbar and Rapp.[2] Intravesical BCG has been approved by the US Food and Drug Administration (FDA) for the treatment of superficial bladder cancer. One of its earliest anticancer uses was in the treatment of melanoma.

Dr Donald Morton[6] was the first to explore this route of treatment. He reported his 7-year experience with 151 patients; 90% of injected lesions and 17% of uninjected lesions regressed. Responding lesions were intradermal, with subcutaneous lesions less likely to respond. Twenty-five percent of the responders remained disease free for between 1 and 6 years. Mastrangelo and colleagues[7] reported a series of 15 patients treated every 2 weeks for a minimum of 5 treatments. There were 2 complete and 3 partial responders. Again, remissions were durable, lasting years to decades.

Storm and colleagues[8] reported a series of patients with recurrent melanoma of the lower extremities treated initially with intralesional BCG. Twenty of 27 patients had complete or transient disease control. Nonresponders and those whose disease eventually progressed were treated with hyperthermic perfusion with L-phenylalanine mustard. Objective responses were seen in 7 of 9 patients. As with most therapies in oncology, a successful single agent is then combined with a second in an attempt to improve response rates. BCG was combined with topical imiquimod, an agent that signals the innate immune system through toll-like receptor-7. Kidner and colleagues[9] treated 9 patients with broad areas of in-transit disease with intralesional BCG followed by topical imiquimod 5 to 7 days a week after an inflammatory response was seen with BCG. Patients were treated until complete remission or progression. Five of 9 patients achieved a complete response (CR) and 3 of the remaining 4 were rendered clinically disease free surgically. All patients were alive at 30 months of follow-up.

Overall, injected nodules disappear 90% of the time and in 20% of patients noninjected regional metastases regress as well.[10] Regression of visceral disease remains elusive but has been reported.[11] Toxicity consists primarily of injection site reactions; the sites most frequently ulcerate and require 6 to 8 weeks to heal. About 2 hours after the injection the patient experiences flulike symptoms that are easily controlled with antipyretics. A BCG bacteremia can occur, resulting in granulomatous changes in the liver and lungs. BCG infections are readily eradicated with isoniazid. The systemic toxicity of BCG is likely related to a transient BCG bacteremia resulting from the intratumoral injection under pressure. This toxicity can be largely avoided by using the scarification approach (discussed later). The systemic toxicity of BCG has been most systematically reported for intravesical use in bladder cancer.[12]

So why is BCG so uncommonly used in clinical practice? A therapy with a 90% response rate is unheard of in most tumor types. We believe it is secondary to a lack of training and exposure to the technique in fellowship. Although intralesional therapy is not unique to melanoma it is most commonly used in this disease, and therefore only trainees at tertiary care institutions with large populations of patients with melanoma would have exposure to this technique. It is not difficult and can be used in any medical oncologist's or oncologic surgeon's office.

MECHANICS OF INJECTING BACILLE CALMETTE-GUERIN

To inject BCG, the first step is the proper selection of target lesions. They should be dermal or cutaneous. As noted earlier, subcutaneous lesions do not respond well because they do not erupt at the surface. Second, the most distal lesions should be injected first, because up to 20% of uninjected lesions in the draining basin respond. Third, they should be in a nonirradiated field because areas of prior irradiated skin do not respond well.

Once the target lesions have been identified, the patient is premedicated with acetaminophen or ibuprofen. The vial of BCG (Merck Sharpe & Dohme, NDC 0005206020) containing 1×10^8 to 8×10^8 organisms (as colony forming units [CFU]) is reconstituted with 1 mL of sterile water. The contents of the vial are then diluted to a total volume of 10 mL of sterile water for a 1:10 dilution ($1–8 \times 10^7$ CFU/mL). One milliliter is then drawn up in a 1-mL Luer Lock syringe with a 25-gauge needle. The selected lesions are cleaned with alcohol and then the needle is inserted from the base of the lesion toward the center. The BCG is then injected slowly. Each lesion should accommodate between 0.05 ($0.5–4 \times 10^6$ CFU) and 0.10 mL ($1–8 \times 10^6$ CFU). Because the solution is under pressure, wait 30 to 60 seconds before withdrawing the needle so that the BCG is not allowed to run out of the lesion.

We typically inject 0.4 to 0.8 mL of the 1:10 dilution of BCG in the first session depending on the number of lesions. Instructions are given to the patient to redose the acetaminophen or ibuprofen every 6 to 8 hours for the first 24 hours. If fever of more than 38.0°C (100.4°F) persists for more than 48 hours we typically consider treatment with isoniazid.

The patient returns for the second treatment in 2 to 3 weeks' time. If there is minimal induration or erythema we continue retreatment at a 1:10 dilution. If they have an intensely suppurative reaction we retreat at a 1:20 dilution and typically inject previously uninjected lesions, again working distal to proximal. This process creates an abscess. The drainage and erythema become intense, because this is what is intended: a large immune reaction (**Fig. 1**).

SCARIFICATION WITH BACILLE CALMETTE-GUERIN

The alternative to intralesional BCG is scarification with BCG, which was described in the 1970s by Richman and colleagues[13] at the MD Anderson Cancer Center. They developed this method to alleviate some the systemic side effects of intralesional BCG. They treated 13 patients by scarification with 3 CRs and 4 partial responses (PRs). We typically reserve this method for broad-based lesions in the dermis that do not present as discrete nodules.

The technique for this method is different. An 18-gauge needle is used to create a grid of superficial cuts through the tumor, just deep enough to create capillary bleeding. The BCG vial is reconstituted with just enough sterile water to create a thick paste. The paste is mixed with the blood on the surface of the lesion and then dried with a hair dryer on the cool setting. The area is wrapped with a plastic cover. We find that a roll from the grocery store works best, and is kept in place for 24 hours. This process is typically repeated every 2 to 4 weeks.

INTERLEUKIN-2

IL-2 is a member of the cytokine family and is necessary for the growth and proliferation of thymic-derived (T cells) lymphocytes to become effector T cells. It was first approved for the systemic treatment of melanoma in 1998, with response rates of 10% to 15 %. Although responses are durable, systemic toxicity (the capillary leak syndrome) hindered its wider acceptance.[14] IL-2 also has been used for intralesional therapy, thus avoiding the treatment-limiting toxicity of systemic administration.

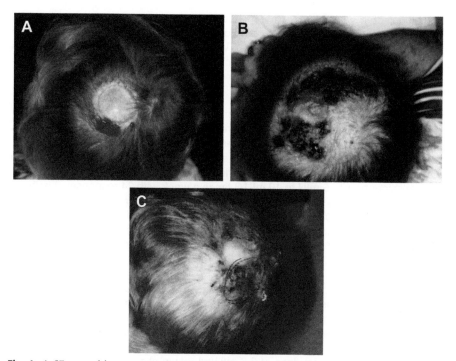

Fig. 1. A 67-year-old woman with multiple local recurrences of a scalp melanoma despite wide excision and skin grafting. She was treated with intralesional BCG from 6/12/12 to 12/9/12 with biopsy-confirmed complete remission. However, she developed metastatic disease involving bone and nodes 6 months later. (*A*) Initiation of therapy. (*B*) 6 weeks after initiation of therapy. (*C*) 3 months after initiation of therapy.

One of the larger single studies of intralesional IL-2 was a series of 39 patients treated by Boyd and colleagues.[15] Patients received biweekly injections for 4 to 7 weeks, with a mean dose of 2.08 mL (5 million units/mL). The investigators noted an overall response rate of 82% with 51% CR and 31% PR. This response was sustained in those who achieved a CR, with 77% of those in CR remaining disease free at 5 years. A similar study by Radny and colleagues[16] of 24 patients showed a response rate of 62.5%.

Byers and colleagues[17] performed a retrospective review of all published reports from intralesional IL-2 for in-transit disease. Their pooled analysis included 140 patients showing a CR in 68 of 140 patients. The dosing varied from 5 days a week every 21 days to the most common frequency of 2 to 3 times a week. Intensity and duration of treatment did not seem to affect the response rate.

The toxicity profile is much improved with intralesional IL-2 as opposed to systemic administration. In particular, capillary leak syndrome has not been observed with intralesional IL-2. The most common side effects include fever, chills, flulike syndrome, and painful swelling and erythema at the injection sites. Most of the systemic symptoms can be alleviated by the pretreatment of the patient with acetaminophen or ibuprofen and continuation of the same for 24 hours after treatment.

The IL-2 injections are performed technically in the same fashion as described for BCG. In our own practice, we reconstitute a vial of 22×10^6 units in a total of 1.0 mL of sterile water, yielding a concentration of 2.2×10^6 units/0.1 mL. Lesions are each injected with 0.1 mL, with up to 6 lesions being injected per session. The larger lesions can receive a larger portion of the total dose. We attempt to treat 2 to 3 times a week for a minimum of 4 weeks. Two to 3 months are required for regression of uninjected lesions. Treated lesions respond more promptly.

INTERFERON

Interferons are glycoproteins used to communicate between cells to eradicate pathogens. They enhance host immunity by upregulating antigen presentation. Interferon has been FDA approved for the systemic treatment of melanoma and renal cell cancer. Both alfa and beta interferon have been studied intralesionally in melanoma. Von Wussow and colleagues[18] reported a series of 51 patients treated with interferon alfa intralesionally with 6 mIU to 10 mIU 3 times a week with 24 responses. Fierlbeck and colleagues[19] had a series of 10 patients treated with interferon beta in doses of 3 mIU or 5 mIU. A 50% response rate was seen at the 5-mIU dose and none at the 3 mIU. When given intralesionally at doses of 1 to 2 mIU/lesion and no more than 5 mIU/session, the profound flulike symptoms that complicate systemic therapy are almost entirely avoided.

Imiquimod and Interleukin-2

The combination of topical imiquimod and IL-2 has also been studied. Green and colleagues[20] treated patients with a total of 182 lesions, both cutaneous and subcutaneous. The overall response rate was 50.5%, with 40.7% comprising a CR. They treated the lesions with topical imiquimod daily for 4 weeks followed by injection of IL-2 3 times a week with a total dose of 3.6 mIU/mL given at each session. The lesions were evaluated for response after 3 months.[16] This CR is lower than that of the pooled analysis; however, the sample size is small.

Garcia and colleagues[21] reported a 100% CR in 3 patients with 64 lesions treated with imiquimod and IL-2. However, the dose of IL-2 was substantially higher than in Green and colleagues'[20] study. Garcia and colleagues[21] used 22 mIU per session as opposed to 3.2 mIU (**Fig. 2**).

GRANULOCYTE-MACROPHAGE COLONY-STIMULATING FACTOR

GM-CSF stimulates hematopoietic stem cells to produce granulocytes and monocytes. The latter migrate into the tissues where they mature into macrophages and dendritic cells, professional antigen-presenting cells that facilitate the initiation of a host immune response. GM-CSF has been injected directly into melanoma metastases with some success. However, its rapid clearance from the injection site requires frequent readministration, which in turn has hampered its implementation. Intralesional GM-CSF is being pursed using viral vectors for more sustained persistence at the injection sites.

To circumvent the issue of rapid dissipation from the injection site, Mastrangelo and colleagues[22] developed a vaccinia/GM-CSF recombinant. Seven patients with dermal and/or subcutaneous metastases were treated with twice-weekly intratumoral injections of escalating doses (10^4 to 2×10^7 plaque-forming units [PFU] per lesion; 10^4 to 8×10^7 PFU/session) of a vaccinia recombinant virus for 6 weeks. Patients with responding or stable disease remained on treatment until tumor resolution or progression. Systemic toxicity was rare, dose dependent, and limited to mild flulike symptoms. Local inflammation, at times with pustule formation, was consistently seen with doses of greater than or equal to 10^7 PFU/lesions. These pustules were less severe and less chronic than those seen with intralesional BCG. All 7 patients

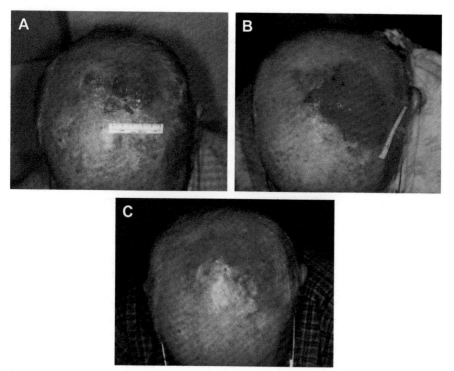

Fig. 2. An 87-year-old man with multiple local recurrences of a scalp melanoma despite repeated surgical excision. Because of his age and comorbid conditions he received topical (imiquimod) and intralesional (IL-2 and GM-CSF) therapy from 09/13/10 to 12/23/10. Treatment sessions totaled 17. He achieved biopsy-confirmed complete remission and remains in complete remission at 44+ months. (*A*) Pretreatment, (*B*) midtreatment, (*C*) posttreatment.

developed an antivaccinia humoral immune response. There were 1 complete, 1 partial, and 3 mixed responses. The 2 patients with the largest tumor burdens did not respond.

GM-CSF has been used most recently as part of an oncolytic herpes virus as intralesional therapy for melanoma. The mechanism of action of this oncolytic virus seems to be 2-fold: direct destruction of tumor cells and stimulation of dendritic cells through the accumulation of GM-CSF, thus inducing tumor-specific immunity. Initially known as Oncvex and now talimogene laherparepvec (TVEC), this agent was shown to have a 26% response rate in both injected and uninjected lesions, including responses in visceral metastasis. This phase II study evaluated 50 patients who received a median of 6 intratumoral injections. The side effects were mild and most commonly included flulike symptoms.[23,24]

The success of this phase 2 study prompted further investigation through a phase III randomized study of patients 2:1 to intralesional TVEC or subcutaneous GM-CSF at 125 μg/m^2 every day for 14 days every 28 days. The primary end point was durable response rate, continuous for greater than 6 months. The interim analysis of 436 patients reported at American Society of Clinical Oncology (ASCO) in June 2013 showed a response rate identical to the phase II study of 26%, with a durable response rate of 16% compared with a response rate of 6% for the GM-CSF arm.[25]

ROSE BENGAL

Rose bengal, a water-soluble xanthene dye, has been shown to induce regression in both injected and uninjected lesions.[26,27] This regression was most recently evaluated in a phase II study reported at ASCO in June 2014. Eighty patients were treated with intralesional rose bengal up to 4 times over a 16-week period and followed for a year. A 51% overall response rate was seen and 26% CR. In a 28-patient subgroup analysis of patients who had all of their lesions injected, a 71% response rate was seen.[28]

It is well tolerated, with symptoms being confined to local reactions.

The mechanism of action seems to be preferential uptake of the rose bengal by tumor cell lysosomes. This uptake causes lysosome rupture and tumor cell necrosis. This necrosis in turn causes a tumor-specific immune response. In preclinical trials an increase in tumor-infiltrating lymphocytes was seen. This systemic immune response is thought to be responsible for the resolution of uninjected lesions.[29]

ALLOVECTIN

Allovectin is different from the previously discussed intralesional agents. It is a plasmid DNA–based immunotherapy composed of a human leukocyte antigen (HLA)-B7/beta2 microglobulin DNA liposome complex.[30] It is thought to have 3 mechanisms of action: the first is inducing a T-cell response against the allogeneic target of HLA-B7, which is expressed in a minority of patients.[31] Second is the induction of a T-cell response against tumor antigens once major histocompatibility complex class I expression is restored by insertion of Beta 2 microglobulin, and induction of immune and inflammatory responses. Although initially encouraging in earlier studies, results of a phase III randomized study did not show statistically significant improvement in the response rate or overall survival when compared with first-line chemotherapy consisting of dacarbazine or temozolomide.[32,33]

DISCUSSION

Overall, agents such as BCG, IL-2, interferon, rose bengal, and GM-CSF/viral recombinants, alone or in combination, are all viable options for treatment of local-regional dermal and subcutaneous melanoma metastases through intralesional injections. Remission rates are significantly higher than when they are used systemically to treat metastatic disease, suggesting that the concentration of the agent within the tumor is a significant factor in determining response. The mechanism of the antitumor effect is postulated to be immunologic but a bystander effect caused by the inflammatory response is also possible. The therapy is well tolerated with much less toxicity then when these agents are used systemically. This approach is especially useful when treating disease in cosmetically or functionally eloquent areas or where the extent of involvement precludes surgical excision. Intralesional therapy should be considered in such circumstances before resorting to systemic therapy. However, the response of nonregional disease is infrequent.

REFERENCES

1. Coley WB. The treatment of malignant tumors by repeated inoculations of Erysipelas, with a report of 10 original cases. Am J Med Sci 1893;105:487–511.
2. Zbar B, Rapp HJ. Immunotherapy of Guinea pig cancer with BCG. Cancer 1974; 34:1532–40.

3. Belisario JC, Milton GW. The experimental local therapy of cutaneous metastases of malignant melanoblastomas with cow pox vaccine or colcemid (Demecolcine or Omaine). Aust J Dermatol 1961;6:113–8.
4. Everall JD, Wand L, O'Doherty CI, et al. Treatment of primary melanoma by intralesional vaccine before excision. Lancet 1975;2:583.
5. Mastrangelo MJ, Maguire HC Jr, McCue PA. A pilot study demonstrating the feasibility of using intratumoral vaccinia injections as a vector for gene transfer. Vaccin Res 1995;4:55–69.
6. Morton DL. Immunotherapy of melanoma. Summary of a 7 year experience. Ann Surg 1974;180:635–43.
7. Mastrangelo MJ, Sulit HL, Prehn LM, et al. Intralesional BCG in the treatment of metastatic melanoma. Cancer 1976;37:684–92.
8. Storm FK, Sparks FC, Morton DL. Treatment of melanoma of the lower extremity with intralesional injection of Bacille Calmette-Guerin and hyperthermic perfusion. Surg Gynecol Obstet 1979;159:17–21.
9. Kidner TB, Morton DL, Lee DJ, et al. Combined intralesional bacille Calmette-Guerin, (BCG) and topical imiquimod for in-transit melanoma. J Immunother 2012;35:716–20.
10. Rosenberg SA, Rapp HJ. Intralesional immunotherapy of melanoma with BCG. Med Clin North Am 1976;60:419–30.
11. Mastrangelo MJ, Bellet RE, Berkelhammer J, et al. Regression of pulmonary metastatic disease associated with intralesional BCG therapy of intracutaneous melanoma metastases. Cancer 1975;36:1305–8.
12. O'Donnell MA. Complications of intravesical BCG immunotherapy. UpToDate. Topic 2973, Version 6.0. 2013.
13. Richman SP, Mavligit GM, Wolk R, et al. Epilesional scarification. JAMA 1975;234:1233–5.
14. Temple-Oberle CF, Byers BA, Hurdle V, et al. Intra-lesional interleukin-2 therapy for in transit melanoma. J Surg Oncol 2014;109:327–31.
15. Boyd KU, Wehrli BM, Temple CL. Intra-lesional interleukin-2 for the treatment of in-transit melanoma. J Surg Oncol 2011;104:711–7.
16. Radny P, Caroli WM, Bauer J, et al. Phase II trial of intralesional therapy with IL-2 in soft tissue melanoma metastases. Br J Cancer 2003;89:1620–6.
17. Byers B, Temple-Oberle CF, McKinnon JG, et al. Treatment of intransit melanoma with intralesional interleukin-2: a systematic review. Can J Plast Surg 2013;24:142.
18. Von Wussow P, Block B, Harmenn F, et al. Intralesional interferon-alpha therapy in advanced malignant melanoma. Cancer 1988;61:1071–4.
19. Fierlbeck G, d'Hoedt B, Stroeble W, et al. Intralesional therapy of melanoma metastases with recombinant interferon-beta. Hautarzt 1992;43:16–21.
20. Green DS, Bodman-Smith AG, Fisher MD. Phase I/II study of topical imiquimod and intralesional interleukin-2 in the treatment of accessible metastases in malignant melanoma. Br J Dermatol 2007;156:337–45.
21. Garcia MS, Ono Y, Martinez SR, et al. Complete regression of subcutaneous and cutaneous metastatic melanoma with high-dose intralesional interleukin 2 in combination with topical imiquimod and retinoid cream. Melanoma Res 2011;21:235–43.
22. Mastrangelo MJ, Maguire HC Jr, Eisenlohr LC, et al. Intratumoral recombinant GM-CSF-encoding virus as gene therapy in patients with cutaneous melanoma. Cancer Gene Ther 1998;5:409–22.
23. Senzer NN, Kaufman HL, Amatruda T, et al. Phase II clinical trial of a granulocyte-macrophage colony-stimulating factor-encoding, second-generation oncolytic

herpesvirus in patients with unresectable metastatic melanoma. J Clin Oncol 2009;27:5763–71.

24. Kaufman HL, Kim DW, DeRaffele G, et al. Local and distant immunity induced by intralesional vaccination with an oncolytic herpes virus encoding GM-CSF in patients with stage IIIc and IV melanoma. Ann Surg Oncol 2010;17:718–30.

25. Andtbacka RH, Colichio FA, Amatruda T, et al. OPTiM: a randomized phase III trial of talimogene laherparepvec (T-VEC) versus subcutaneous (SC) granulocyte-macrophage colony-stimulating factor (GM-CSF) for the treatment of unresected stage IIIB/C and IV melanoma. J Clin Oncol 2013;31 [abstract: LBA 9008].

26. Toomey P, Kodumudi K, Weber A, et al. Intralesional injection of Rose Bengal induces a systemic tumor-specific immune response in murine models of melanoma and breast cancer. PLoS One 2013;8(7):e68561.

27. Thompson JF, Hersey P, Wachter E. Chemoablation of metastatic melanoma using intralesion Rose Bengal. Melanoma Res 2008;18:405–11.

28. Ross MI. Intralesional therapy with PV-10 (Rose Bengal) for in-transit melanoma. J Surg Oncol 2014;109:314–9.

29. Agarwala SS, Thompson JF, Smithers BM, et al. Efficacy of intralesional Rose Bengal in patients receiving injection of all existing melanoma in phase II study of PV 10-MM-02. J Clin Oncol 2014 [abstract: 9027].

30. Bedkian AY, Richards J, Kharkevitch D, et al. A phase 2 study of high-dose allovectin-7 in patients with advanced metastatic melanoma. Melanoma Res 2010; 20:218–26.

31. Doukas J, Rolland A. Mechanisms of action underlying the immunotherapeutic activity of Allovectin in advanced melanoma. Cancer Gene Ther 2012;19:811–7.

32. Leach B. Allovectin falters in late stage melanoma trial. 2013. Available at: Onclive.com. Accessed July 30, 2014.

33. Stopeck A. Transfer of allovectin-7 an HLA-B7/B2 microglobulin DNA liposome complex in patients with metastatic melanoma. Clin Cancer Res 2001;7:2285.

Regional Therapies for In-transit Disease

Paul J. Speicher, MD[a], Claire H. Meriwether, BA[a], Douglas S. Tyler, MD[*,b]

KEYWORDS

- In-transit melanoma • Regional therapy • Isolated limb infusion
- Isolated limb perfusion

KEY POINTS

- In-transit disease is a challenging pattern of recurrence to manage, occurring in up to 10% of patients with melanoma.
- Regional therapy, by isolated limb infusion or hyperthermic isolated limb perfusion, offers treatment options for patients with nonresectable disease.
- Regional therapies are generally well tolerated, and offer complete response rates of 25% to 50%, although long-term responses are often not durable.
- Future management of in-transit melanoma is likely to involve combination therapies, joining cytotoxic regional therapy and systemic immune-modulating drugs such as anti–cytotoxic T-lymphocyte antigen 4 (CTLA-4) and anti-programmed cell death 1 surface protein molecule agents.

INTRODUCTION

In-transit melanoma occurs in up to 10% of patients with melanoma, and is a pattern of recurrence that presents unique management challenges and opportunities for treatment. In-transit disease is defined as tumor deposits that usually occur somewhere between the primary lesion and its draining regional lymph node basin.[1,2] Although often associated with distant metastases, the presence of in-transit disease is an independent adverse prognostic factor. Unique treatment modalities, in the form of regional chemotherapy, are often necessary because this pattern of recurrent disease is often not amenable to surgical resection.

BACKGROUND
Incidence

In-transit disease is uncommon, occurring in less than 10% of patients diagnosed with melanoma and accounting for 12% to 22% of melanoma recurrences. The presence

[a] Department of Surgery, Duke University Medical Center, 2301 Erwin Road, Durham, NC 27710, USA; [b] Department of Surgery, University of Texas Medical Branch, 301 University Boulevard, Galveston, TX 77555, USA
* Corresponding author. Department of Surgery, 6.146 John Seeley Annex, 301 University Boulevard, Galveston, TX 77555.
E-mail address: doug.tyler@duke.edu

Surg Oncol Clin N Am 24 (2015) 309–322
http://dx.doi.org/10.1016/j.soc.2014.12.008
1055-3207/15/$ – see front matter Published by Elsevier Inc.

surgonc.theclinics.com

of positive nodal disease significantly increases the risk of developing in-transit disease, with estimates suggesting risks as high as 31% when at least 3 positive nodes are present.[3] Although initial disease stage seems to be the most important factor in predicting in-transit recurrences, lesion location may also play a role, with higher rates in the lower extremities versus upper extremities. Early observations also suggested an association between surgical lymphadenectomy and the development of in-transit disease, presumably caused by lymphatic trapping in which outflow obstruction of the draining lymphatic system led to stasis and trapping of tumor deposits. However, in recent larger studies, neither lymphadenectomy nor sentinel lymph node biopsy were associated with an increased risk of developing in-transit metastases.[4–7]

Biology

Although the true underlying biology of in-transit melanoma is unknown, it is thought to be related to small tumor emboli disseminating along the path of lymphatic drainage from the primary tumor to its draining nodal basin. These migrating tumor cells are thought to become ensnared in the draining dermal and subdermal lymphatics, eventually progressing to clinically detectable lesions. Although tumor deposits becoming trapped along the lymphatic drainage remains the most likely biological explanation, other mechanisms have been suggested, including hematogenous spread, similar to that of distant metastases.[8,9] Supporters of this alternative theory argue that, if the lymphatic concept is true, wider margins during primary excision would be expected to include a higher proportion of trapped occult cells and lead to superior clinical outcomes, which is not consistent with current observations. However, the hematogenous theory is not supported by the significant differences in long-term survival observed for patients with stage III versus stage IV disease.

Nomenclature

Several different terms have been used in the literature to describe what is likely to be the same underlying oncologic process. In the past, terms such as satellitosis, locoregional recurrence, and in-transit disease have each been used to describe various clinical findings. Satellitosis was usually defined as a locoregional recurrence that was located within either 2 cm of the excision scar or 5 cm of the initial lesion, whereas the term in-transit disease was reserved for a recurrence occurring at greater distances from the initial lesion or scar. Because such lesions all likely reflect tumor deposits proliferating along paths of lymphatic drainage, it has more recently become apparent that distance from the primary lesion to the site of locoregional recurrence does not carry meaningful prognostic value.[10–13] Consequently, the most recent American Joint Committee on Cancer (AJCC) staging system for melanoma does not distinguish between traditional satellitosis and in-transit lesions, with both being designated as N2 or N3 disease, depending on regional node status.[14] To address the ongoing ambiguity arising from nomenclature issues, many authorities no longer use the term satellitosis, instead referring to all regional nonnodal metastatic disease as in-transit melanoma.

PATIENT EVALUATION OVERVIEW
Presentation

By definition, in-transit melanoma represents locoregionally advanced disease, and is typically discovered months to years after the initial surgical excision of the primary lesion, with a disease-free interval to recurrence ranging from 12 to 16 months.[15,16]

The clinical presentation usually involves from 1 to more than 100 small subcutaneous or cutaneous nodules, although it can be variable (**Fig. 1**). Individual lesions can range from submillimeter to multiple centimeters in diameter, and may take the form of superficial cutaneous (also called epidermotropic) or deeper subcutaneous nodules. For disease located in an extremity, the lesions are often clustered in proximity to the primary lesion, but can also involve the entire extremity extending from the primary tumor to its regional lymphatic basin. For truncal disease, the pattern of distribution can be even more inconsistent, with potentially extensive tumor burden depending on the location of the primary melanoma.

Evaluation

The work-up of patients with in-transit melanoma starts with a thorough skin examination, and in patients with an unclear diagnosis and suspicious lesions it is our practice to use a 3-mm to 5-mm punch biopsy for small superficial lesions and fine-needle aspiration biopsy for larger lesions to obtain pathologic confirmation of melanoma. All major nodal basins should be examined for the presence of clinically involved nodes, and preoperative cross-sectional imaging should be performed to evaluate for distant metastatic spread. In patients who have disease isolated to an extremity and are candidates for general anesthesia, regional chemotherapy should be considered as a first-line therapy.

Dosing

Drug doses for regional therapy are typically based on limb volume, either measured directly or imputed. For hyperthermic isolated limb perfusions (HILPs), melphalan

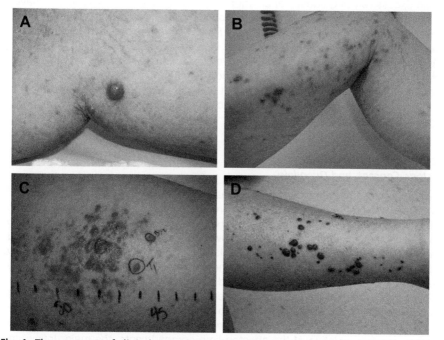

Fig. 1. The spectrum of clinical presentation for patients with in-transit melanoma of the extremity. Disease can manifest as (*A*) low-volume disease or solitary nodules, (*B*) multifocal unpigmented lesions, (*C*) multifocal disease with diffuse dermal spread, or (*D*) traditional multifocal dark pigmented lesions.

doses of 10 mg/L for the lower limb and 13 mg/L for the upper limb are typically used.[17] For isolated limb infusion (ILI), slightly lower doses are used; typically 7.5 mg/L for the lower limb and 10 mg/L for the lower limb, both usually with the addition of 50 to 100 μg/L of actinomycin-D.[18,19]

Multiple techniques to determine the optimal dose for regional therapy have been developed, with the simplest methods relying on patient body weight and/or ideal body weight, offering simple and fast calculations.[20] In recent years such techniques have largely been abandoned, because they have been shown to produce substantial variability compared with more accurate limb volume measurements.[21,22] The original methods described by Wieberdink and colleagues[23] for estimating limb volume relied on a method of measuring water displacement from the submerged limb. Although accurate and still used, this method is hampered by logistical issues related to the nature of the water reservoir apparatus.

An alternative method that has more recently gained popularity is calculation based on limb circumference. In this approach, circumference measurements are taken at standardized intervals (usually 1.5 cm) along the length of the extremity. By calculating the volume of each theoretic slice based on the limb circumference at that level, and summing across the limb, highly accurate estimates of limb volume can be obtained.[22,24] This method offers distinct advantages compared with water displacement techniques, in that it is inexpensive, does not require specialized equipment or facilities, and can be performed at the bedside and on immobile or otherwise functionally impaired individuals.

Although numerous techniques for limb volume calculation have been described, further adjustment is often required, particularly in the setting of obesity in order to avoid excessively large doses of chemotherapy being delivered to limbs that have a disproportionately large amount of fat. Although there remains some debate regarding the role of weight-based dose adjustment for ILI,[25] in our experience, multiplying the calculated limb volume by the quotient of ideal body weight (IBW) and actual body weight to obtain an IBW-adjusted limb volume has helped minimize unnecessary toxicity without compromising clinical response.[24] Furthermore, recent work by Podleska and colleagues[22] has confirmed that this method gives lean limb volume estimates that correlate extremely well with no-fat computed tomography scans, which digitally subtract subcutaneous fat tissue.

REGIONAL CHEMOTHERAPY
History, Concept, and Overview

The origins of limb infusion can be traced back to 1950, when Klopp and colleagues[26] discovered that intra-arterial infusion of nitrogen mustards proved substantially more effective than intravenous administration. However, it was not until 1958 that Creech and colleagues[27] first described what is now considered limb perfusion, adopting advances in cardiopulmonary bypass to isolate and oxygenate the relevant area and administer high-dose intra-arterial chemotherapy. A decade later, Stehlin[28] added hyperthermia to the treatment, with improved results.

The fundamental concept of regional chemotherapy for in-transit melanoma entails vascular isolation of the affected limb, followed by high-dose chemotherapy delivery at doses up to 20 times larger than can be tolerated systemically. Because regional therapy requires isolation of the affected limb compartments, the major inflow and outflow vessels to the area of interest must be accessed and cannulated, and the treatment region must then be completely isolated from the systemic circulation, usually by means of a pneumatic or Esmarch tourniquet. The 2 general approaches to accomplishing this are HILP and ILI. Although both procedures involve regional delivery of high-dose chemotherapy, they differ in several important technical and conceptual aspects.

Isolated Limb Perfusion

HILP as originally described by Creech and colleagues[27] is performed under general anesthesia, and requires exposure and direct cannulation of the vasculature supplying the affected limb. An oncologic regional lymphadenectomy is typically performed concurrently, which has the added benefit of aiding vascular exposure, particularly when accessing the iliac vessels. A proximal tourniquet is then placed, and perfusion is initiated via the cannulated vessels, using a standard extracorporeal bypass circuit with membrane oxygenation to maintain physiologic limb oxygen tension and acid-base status (**Fig. 2**). To achieve hyperthermia with a goal of 40°C, the circuit is heated and external warming blankets are placed on the involved limb. Chemotherapy is typically perfused through the limb circuit for 60 minutes, followed by a washout period of 20 to 30 minutes with crystalloids to facilitate removal of the cytotoxic agents. During the perfusion portion of the procedure, leakage of perfusate into the systemic circulation can pose substantial risks of toxicity, particularly when high-dose tumor necrosis factor alpha (TNF-α) is used in conjunction with cytotoxic therapy. In the past, such leakage was monitored by injecting intravenous fluorescein into the perfusion circuit, and watching for evidence of staining proximal to the tourniquet. More recently, administration of a radiolabeled tracer into the HILP circuit with continuous monitoring of systemic radiation exposure using a precordial gamma probe has provided a more precise method of leak detection. At the conclusion of the procedure, the cannulas are removed, the blood vessels repaired, the tourniquet is removed, and a careful vascular and musculoskeletal examination is performed.

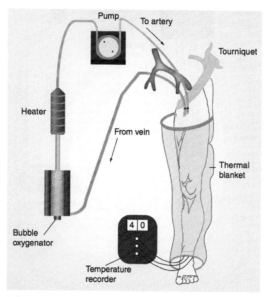

Fig. 2. HILP. (*From* Coleman A, Augustine CK, Beasley G, et al. Optimizing regional infusion treatment strategies for melanoma of the extremities. Expert Rev Anticancer Ther 2009;9(11):1600; with permission.)

Isolated Limb Infusion

ILI was first described by Thompson and colleagues[29] in the mid-1990s as a less-invasive alternative to HILP. During ILI, the target limb vessels are cannulated using percutaneously placed catheters inserted with the aid of fluoroscopy. Similar to HILP, the limb is isolated using an external tourniquet, and is then wrapped in heating blankets. In contrast with HILP, ILI is performed without extracorporeal perfusion and oxygenation, and the perfusate is manually circulated using a syringe and 3-way stop-cock (**Fig. 3**). As a result, the limb becomes markedly acidotic and hypoxic during the procedure, which some clinicians have suggested augments the effectiveness of the melphalan chemotherapy.[30] Although warming blankets and a heat exchanger are typically used, limb temperatures observed during ILI are typically lower than those seen during HILP, and often do not exceed 38.5°C to 39.0°C.[19,31]

One of the primary benefits of ILI compared with HILP is the simplicity and substantially less-invasive nature of the procedure. The infusion of chemotherapy is typically maintained for 30 minutes, followed by washout with crystalloid in a similar manner to HILP. Melphalan doses are often lower than those used in HILP, and treatment-associated morbidity is substantially less, particularly severe morbidity. As a result, ILI can be offered to patients with higher comorbidity burdens and who might not tolerate the more invasive groin exposure required for HILP. Similarly, because of its

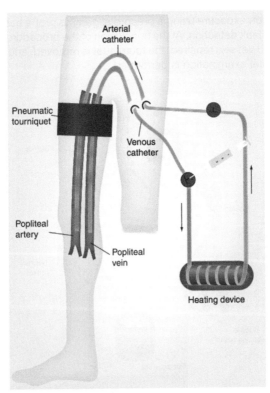

Fig. 3. ILI. (*From* Coleman A, Augustine CK, Beasley G, et al. Optimizing regional infusion treatment strategies for melanoma of the extremities. Expert Rev Anticancer Ther 2009;9(11):1602; with permission.)

less-invasive nature, ILI can be offered as salvage therapy and repeated in situations of treatment failure or recurrent disease. As a result, repeat ILI can be an integral component in the management of recurrent or progressive in-transit disease following failure of initial regional therapy. Although some clinicians have proposed intentionally leveraging this advantage and using ILI as a means of delivering fractionated chemotherapy over the course of multiple treatments, this has not been shown to improve survival compared with single full-dose ILI.[32]

Drugs and Dosing

For any therapeutic agent to be considered for regional therapy, it must not require metabolic transformation to take on a biologically active form. Melphalan has long been established as the primary chemotherapy choice for HILP and ILI. Melphalan is an alkylating agent derived from phenylalanine, which plays a key role in melanin synthesis and is preferentially taken up by melanocytes. Because of this, melphalan has the theoretic advantage of producing selective toxicity in melanin-containing melanoma cells. Systemically, the effective dose of melphalan has been found to exceed the maximally tolerated dose, limiting use as a systemic agent. In contrast, the effective dose is easily achieved with regional therapy, without associated systemic toxicity.

Several other agents have been used, either instead of or in combination with melphalan, for regional therapy treatment of in-transit melanoma. Cisplatin showed significant potential in preclinical studies, and early clinical reports revealed promising response rates, but further developments were limited by concerns over limb-threatening toxicity.[33–37] Similarly, TNF-α held early promise, particularly when combined with interferon-gamma, but widespread use of TNF-α has been limited because of significant concerns over toxicity.[38] When combined with melphalan, TNF-α was effective in preclinical models, but the 2006 ACOSOG (American College of Surgeons Oncology Group) Z0020 trial was terminated early after interim analysis confirmed significantly increased toxicity with the combination therapy without any improvement in clinical response compared with melphalan alone.[39] Temozolomide is a newer alkylating agent that is closely related to melphalan and does not require hepatic conversion to take on an active form. Early results in preclinical animal models of regional therapy showed superior results compared with melphalan.[40] A recently completed multicenter (Duke, Moffitt, and MD Anderson) phase I clinical trial was able to define the maximally tolerated dose of intra-arterial temozolomide in patients with regionally advanced melanoma of the extremity and showed that some patients who did not respond to ILI with melphalan could achieve a complete response to ILI with temozolomide (**Fig. 4**) (Beasley and colleagues,[41] in press).

TREATMENT COMPLICATIONS

Some degree of tissue toxicity is typically seen following regional therapy, presumably because of the high concentration of cytotoxic agents administered. Numerous different grading systems have been proposed to standardize toxicity reporting following treatment. Of these, the most commonly used is that developed by Wieberdink and colleagues,[23] wherein toxicity scores range from grade I, or no evidence of any adverse reaction, to grade V, representing a severe and potentially limb-threatening reaction (**Table 1**). Although in larger series up to 85% of patients experienced grade I to II toxicity, less than 1% of patients experienced grade V toxicity.[42] Although the overall range of toxicity is similar for ILI and HILP, the latter carries a higher risk of higher-grade toxicity, including risk of possible limb loss. Although

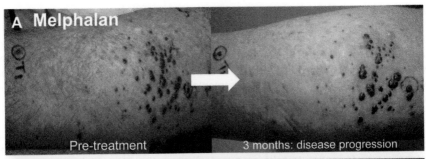

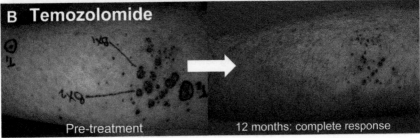

Fig. 4. A complete durable response following temozolomide ILI in a patient who previously progressed after melphalan ILI. (*A*) Progressive disease within 3 months following initial treatment with melphalan ILI. (*B*) The same patient showing complete pathologic response following a subsequent temozolomide ILI, with evidence of residual nonmalignant pigmentation out to 12 months after infusion.

limb loss is rare, with rates ranging from 0.3% for ILI to 2% for HILP, severe muscle toxicity and the development of compartment syndrome necessitating fasciotomy is uncommon but well described, occurring in about 5% of patients depending on how melphalan is dosed. Despite these risks, for both HILP and ILI, most adverse reactions are temporary, often resolving within the first month after surgery.

Strategies to Minimize Complications

Numerous strategies have been developed to reduce the risk of complications associated with regional therapy, in addition to IBW-adjusted dosing as discussed previously. For patients with disease located proximally on the limb, treatment of the

Table 1 Wieberdink toxicity grading scale for severity of complications following regional therapy	
Grade I	No subjective or objective evidence of reaction
Grade II	Slight erythema and/or edema of limb
Grade III	Considerable erythema and/or edema of limb with some blistering; slightly disturbed motility/mobility
Grade IV	Extensive epidermolysis and/or obvious deep tissue damage, causing definite functional disturbances; threatening or manifest compartment syndrome
Grade V	Reaction that may necessitate amputation/limb loss

Adapted from Wieberdink J, Benckhuysen C, Braat RP, et al. Dosimetry in isolation perfusion of the limbs by assessment of perfused tissue volume and grading of toxic tissue reactions. Eur J Cancer Clin Oncol 1982;18:908; with permission.

hand or foot is often not required from an oncologic perspective. In such cases, a second tourniquet can be applied to the wrist or ankle, respectively, to exclude the distalmost portion of the extremity from exposure to chemotherapy. Exclusion of the hand or foot from the circuit can substantially reduce treatment-related morbidity to these areas, which are particularly prone to skin and neurologic toxicities.[43] After surgery, limb elevation may help reduce edema and allow more accurate clinical assessment of limb compartments. It is our practice to measure daily serum creatine kinase (CK) levels to monitor for early evidence of significant muscle toxicity, and to prophylactically administer systemic steroids if CK levels exceed 1000 µg/L. Although CK levels can be informative and raise suspicion, the diagnosis of compartment syndrome and need for urgent fasciotomy are based primarily on careful clinical examination. In some cases, muscle compartment pressures can be measured directly with a handheld intracompartmental pressure monitor, and prove useful in situations in which clinical examination is difficult or unclear.

EVALUATION OF OUTCOME

Reports of outcomes following HILP are widely variable, likely reflecting diverse patient populations and adjunctive treatment strategies, but responses to regional therapy are typically seen within 6 to 12 weeks (**Figs. 5** and **6**). Although single-center studies have described complete response rates of 39% to 82% and overall response rates of 81% to 100%,[44–49] the multicenter ACOSOG Z0020 study reported complete response rates of only 25%.[39] Furthermore, responses are often not durable, with 50% to 60% recurrence rates in the first year and overall 5-year survival of 30% to 40%.[50] Compared with HILP, outcomes following ILI are generally inferior, with complete response rates of 23% to 44% and overall responses of 43% to 100%.[19,31,47,51–54] In comparing patterns of recurrence, ILI has been associated with significantly shorter time to first recurrence (8 months vs 23 months) and an overall higher probability of recurrence (85% vs 65%) compared with HILP.[55] Despite these differences, to date no significant differences in overall survival have been identified between the two treatment approaches.

FUTURE DIRECTIONS AND LONG-TERM RECOMMENDATIONS

Although regional therapy has been established for management of extremity in-transit melanoma for several decades, recent advances in immune modulation may have implications for future treatment of locoregionally advanced disease. Immune checkpoint blockade, via anti–CTLA-4 and anti-PD-1, has generated considerable interest in recent years as a potential therapy for advanced melanoma. Responses that are clinically meaningful may be linked to immune activation, and a growing body of

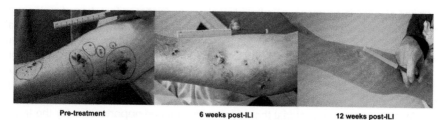

Pre-treatment   6 weeks post-ILI   12 weeks post-ILI

Fig. 5. Typical time course of a complete response following regional therapy, showing steady resolution of in-transit melanoma lesions over a 12-week postoperative period.

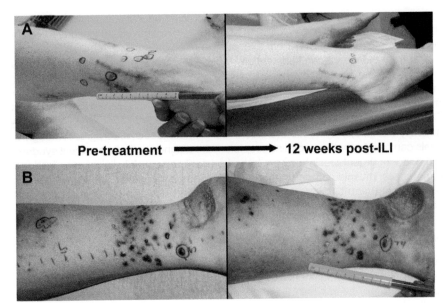

Fig. 6. Patterns of tumor regression in 2 patients who experienced complete responses following regional therapy. Nonpigmented lesions (A) typically resolve visually, whereas pigmented lesions (B) following complete response often leave a tattooed-appearing area consisting of pigment-laden macrophages with no viable tumor on biopsy.

evidence suggests that therapeutic responses may be linked to immune activation.[56–60] Regional therapy itself has been shown to generate an immune response, which may work in concert with cytotoxic chemotherapy to generate a tumor response.

In light of these advances, clinical trials exploring the role of immune activation with ipilimumab, a human IgG1-kappa monoclonal antibody to CTLA-4, in combination with cytotoxic regional chemotherapy have already started. Specifically, a trial investigating the role of adjuvant ipilimumab administered following melphalan ILI is currently enrolling patients at Memorial Sloane Kettering Cancer Center (clinicaltrials.gov: NCT01323517). Similarly, a multicenter trial based at Duke University exploring neoadjuvant ipilimumab before melphalan ILI is expected to begin enrolling patients by the end of 2014 (clinicaltrials.gov: NCT02115243).

SUMMARY

In-transit disease is an uncommon but clinically important manifestation of melanoma recurrence, and often allows unique treatment opportunities in the form of regional therapy. Over the past half-century, numerous advances in regional therapy have been made, including HILP and ILI. With recent innovations in immune manipulation and checkpoint blockade for the treatment of locally advanced and metastatic disease, future applications of regional therapy are likely to involve combination therapy with cytotoxic agents and novel immune modulators. Despite this changing landscape in melanoma treatment, regional therapy provides unique opportunities for the treatment of unresectable disease, and offers a unique platform for investigation of novel therapeutics in early-stage clinical trials.

REFERENCES

1. Meier F, Will S, Ellwanger U, et al. Metastatic pathways and time courses in the orderly progression of cutaneous melanoma. Br J Dermatol 2002;147:62–70.
2. Pawlik TM, Ross MI, Johnson MM, et al. Predictors and natural history of in-transit melanoma after sentinel lymphadenectomy. Ann Surg Oncol 2005;12:587–96.
3. Cascinelli N, Bufalino R, Marolda R, et al. Regional non-nodal metastases of cutaneous melanoma. Eur J Surg Oncol 1986;12:175–80.
4. Kang JC, Wanek LA, Essner R, et al. Sentinel lymphadenectomy does not increase the incidence of in-transit metastases in primary melanoma. J Clin Oncol 2005;23:4764–70.
5. Morton DL, Thompson JF, Cochran AJ, et al. Sentinel-node biopsy or nodal observation in melanoma. N Engl J Med 2006;355:1307–17.
6. Pawlik TM, Ross MI, Thompson JF, et al. The risk of in-transit melanoma metastasis depends on tumor biology and not the surgical approach to regional lymph nodes. J Clin Oncol 2005;23:4588–90.
7. van Poll D, Thompson JF, Colman MH, et al. A sentinel node biopsy does not increase the incidence of in-transit metastasis in patients with primary cutaneous melanoma. Ann Surg Oncol 2005;12:597–608.
8. Griffiths RW, Briggs JC. Incidence of locally metastatic ('recurrent') cutaneous malignant melanoma following conventional wide margin excisional surgery for invasive clinical stage I tumours: importance of maximal primary tumour thickness. Br J Surg 1986;73:349–53.
9. Heenan PJ, Ghaznawie M. The pathogenesis of local recurrence of melanoma at the primary excision site. Br J Plast Surg 1999;52:209–13.
10. Häffner AC, Garbe C, Burg G, et al. The prognosis of primary and metastasising melanoma. An evaluation of the TNM classification in 2,495 patients. Br J Cancer 1992;66:856–61.
11. Karakousis CP, Temple DF, Moore R, et al. Prognostic parameters in recurrent malignant melanoma. Cancer 1983;52:575–9.
12. Roses DF, Karp NS, Oratz R, et al. Survival with regional and distant metastases from cutaneous malignant melanoma. Surg Gynecol Obstet 1991;172:262–8.
13. Singletary SE, Tucker SL, Boddie AW. Multivariate analysis of prognostic factors in regional cutaneous metastases of extremity melanoma. Cancer 1988;61:1437–40.
14. Balch CM, Gershenwald JE, Soong SJ, et al. Final version of 2009 AJCC melanoma staging and classification. J Clin Oncol 2009;27:6199–206.
15. Lee YT. Loco-regional primary and recurrent melanoma: III. Update of natural history and non-systemic treatments (1980-1987). Cancer Treat Rev 1988;15:135–62.
16. Wong JH, Cagle LA, Kopald KH, et al. Natural history and selective management of in transit melanoma. J Surg Oncol 1990;44:146–50.
17. Eggermont AM, Schraffordt Koops H, Liénard D, et al. Isolated limb perfusion with high-dose tumor necrosis factor-alpha in combination with interferon-gamma and melphalan for nonresectable extremity soft tissue sarcomas: a multi-center trial. J Clin Oncol 1996;14:2653–65.
18. Coleman A, Augustine CK, Beasley G, et al. Optimizing regional infusion treatment strategies for melanoma of the extremities. Expert Rev Anticancer Ther 2009;9:1599–609.
19. Lindnér P, Doubrovsky A, Kam PC, et al. Prognostic factors after isolated limb infusion with cytotoxic agents for melanoma. Ann Surg Oncol 2002;9:127–36.

20. Byrne DS, McKay AJ, Blackie R, et al. A comparison of dosimetric methods in isolated limb perfusion with melphalan for malignant melanoma of the lower extremity. Eur J Cancer 1996;32A:2082–7.

21. Pai MP. Drug dosing based on weight and body surface area: mathematical assumptions and limitations in obese adults. Pharmacotherapy 2012;32:856–68.

22. Podleska LE, Poeppel T, Herbrik M, et al. Drug dosage in isolated limb perfusion: evaluation of a limb volume model for extremity volume calculation. World J Surg Oncol 2014;12:81.

23. Wieberdink J, Benckhuysen C, Braat RP, et al. Dosimetry in isolation perfusion of the limbs by assessment of perfused tissue volume and grading of toxic tissue reactions. Eur J Cancer Clin Oncol 1982;18:905–10.

24. McMahon N, Cheng TY, Beasley GM, et al. Optimizing melphalan pharmacokinetics in regional melanoma therapy: does correcting for ideal body weight alter regional response or toxicity? Ann Surg Oncol 2009;16:953–61.

25. Huismans AM, Kroon HM, Haydu LE, et al. Is melphalan dose adjustment according to ideal body weight useful in isolated limb infusion for melanoma? Ann Surg Oncol 2012;19:3050–6.

26. Barberio R, Berry N, Bateman J, et al. Combined administration of aureomycin and nitrogen mustard. Effects of the intra-arterial administration on human cancer. Cancer 1953;6:280–7.

27. Creech O, Krementz ET, Ryan RF, et al. Chemotherapy of cancer: regional perfusion utilizing an extracorporeal circuit. Ann Surg 1958;148:616–32.

28. Stehlin JS. Hyperthermic perfusion with chemotherapy for cancers of the extremities. Surg Gynecol Obstet 1969;129:305–8.

29. Thompson JF, Kam PC, Waugh RC, et al. Isolated limb infusion with cytotoxic agents: a simple alternative to isolated limb perfusion. Semin Surg Oncol 1998; 14:238–47.

30. Siemann DW, Chapman M, Beikirch A. Effects of oxygenation and pH on tumor cell response to alkylating chemotherapy. Int J Radiat Oncol Biol Phys 1991;20:287–9.

31. Beasley GM, Petersen RP, Yoo J, et al. Isolated limb infusion for in-transit malignant melanoma of the extremity: a well-tolerated but less effective alternative to hyperthermic isolated limb perfusion. Ann Surg Oncol 2008;15:2195–205.

32. Lindnér P, Thompson JF, De Wilt JH, et al. Double isolated limb infusion with cytotoxic agents for recurrent and metastatic limb melanoma. Eur J Surg Oncol 2004; 30:433–9.

33. Aigner K, Hild P, Henneking K, et al. Regional perfusion with cis-platinum and dacarbazine. Recent Results Cancer Res 1983;86:239–45.

34. Roseman JM. Effective management of extremity cancers using cisplatin and etoposide in isolated limb perfusions. J Surg Oncol 1987;35:170–2.

35. Santinami M, Belli F, Cascinelli N, et al. Seven years experience with hyperthermic perfusions in extracorporeal circulation for melanoma of the extremities. J Surg Oncol 1989;42:201–8.

36. Thompson JF, Gianoutsos MP. Isolated limb perfusion for melanoma: effectiveness and toxicity of cisplatin compared with that of melphalan and other drugs. World J Surg 1992;16:227–33.

37. Wile AG, Guilmette E, Friedberg H, et al. A model of experimental isolation perfusion using cis-platinum. J Surg Oncol 1982;21:37–41.

38. Fraker DL, Alexander HR, Andrich M, et al. Treatment of patients with melanoma of the extremity using hyperthermic isolated limb perfusion with melphalan, tumor necrosis factor, and interferon gamma: results of a tumor necrosis factor dose-escalation study. J Clin Oncol 1996;14:479–89.

39. Cornett WR, McCall LM, Petersen RP, et al. Randomized multicenter trial of hyper-thermic isolated limb perfusion with melphalan alone compared with melphalan plus tumor necrosis factor: American College of Surgeons Oncology Group Trial Z0020. J Clin Oncol 2006;24:4196–201.

40. Ueno T, Ko SH, Grubbs E, et al. Modulation of chemotherapy resistance in regional therapy: a novel therapeutic approach to advanced extremity melanoma using intra-arterial temozolomide in combination with systemic O6-benzylgua-nine. Mol Cancer Ther 2006;5:732–8.

41. Beasley GM, Speicher PJ, Augustine CK, et al. A multicenter phase I dose esca-lation trial to evaluate the Safety and tolerability of intra-arterial temozolomide for patients with advanced extremity melanoma using normothermic isolated limb infusion. Annals of Surgical Oncology 2015;22:287–94.

42. Klaase JM, Kroon BB, van Geel BN, et al. Patient- and treatment-related factors associated with acute regional toxicity after isolated perfusion for melanoma of the extremities. Am J Surg 1994;167:618–20.

43. Padussis JC, Steerman SN, Tyler DS, et al. Pharmacokinetics & drug resistance of melphalan in regional chemotherapy: ILP versus ILI. Int J Hyperthermia 2008; 24:239–49.

44. Aloia TA, Grubbs E, Onaitis M, et al. Predictors of outcome after hyperthermic iso-lated limb perfusion: role of tumor response. Arch Surg 2005;140:1115–20.

45. Di Filippo F, Calabrò A, Giannarelli D, et al. Prognostic variables in recurrent limb melanoma treated with hyperthermic antiblastic perfusion. Cancer 1989;63: 2551–61.

46. Minor DR, Allen RE, Alberts D, et al. A clinical and pharmacokinetic study of iso-lated limb perfusion with heat and melphalan for melanoma. Cancer 1985;55: 2638–44.

47. Raymond AK, Beasley GM, Broadwater G, et al. Current trends in regional ther-apy for melanoma: lessons learned from 225 regional chemotherapy treatments between 1995 and 2010 at a single institution. J Am Coll Surg 2011;213:306–16.

48. Sanki A, Kam PC, Thompson JF. Long-term results of hyperthermic, isolated limb perfusion for melanoma: a reflection of tumor biology. Ann Surg 2007;245:591–6.

49. Storm FK, Morton DL. Value of therapeutic hyperthermic limb perfusion in advanced recurrent melanoma of the lower extremity. Am J Surg 1985;150:32–5.

50. Grünhagen DJ, Brunstein F, Graveland WJ, et al. One hundred consecutive iso-lated limb perfusions with TNF-alpha and melphalan in melanoma patients with multiple in-transit metastases. Ann Surg 2004;240:939–47 [discussion: 947–8].

51. Beasley GM, Caudle A, Petersen RP, et al. A multi-institutional experience of iso-lated limb infusion: defining response and toxicity in the US. J Am Coll Surg 2009; 208:706–15 [discussion: 715–7].

52. Brady MS, Brown K, Patel A, et al. A phase II trial of isolated limb infusion with melphalan and dactinomycin for regional melanoma and soft tissue sarcoma of the extremity. Ann Surg Oncol 2006;13:1123–9.

53. Kroon HM, Moncrieff M, Kam PC, et al. Outcomes following isolated limb infusion for melanoma. A 14-year experience. Ann Surg Oncol 2008;15:3003–13.

54. Mian R, Henderson MA, Speakman D, et al. Isolated limb infusion for melanoma: a simple alternative to isolated limb perfusion. Can J Surg 2001;44:189–92.

55. Sharma K, Beasley G, Turley R, et al. Patterns of recurrence following complete response to regional chemotherapy for in-transit melanoma. Ann Surg Oncol 2012;19:2563–71.

56. Abastado JP. The next challenge in cancer immunotherapy: controlling T-cell traffic to the tumor. Cancer Res 2012;72:2159–61.

57. Boni A, Cogdill AP, Dang P, et al. Selective BRAFV600E inhibition enhances T-cell recognition of melanoma without affecting lymphocyte function. Cancer Res 2010;70:5213–9.

58. Hong M, Puaux AL, Huang C, et al. Chemotherapy induces intratumoral expression of chemokines in cutaneous melanoma, favoring T-cell infiltration and tumor control. Cancer Res 2011;71:6997–7009.

59. Nardin A, Wong WC, Tow C, et al. Dacarbazine promotes stromal remodeling and lymphocyte infiltration in cutaneous melanoma lesions. J Invest Dermatol 2011; 131:1896–905.

60. Prescott DM, Charles HC, Poulson JM, et al. The relationship between intracellular and extracellular pH in spontaneous canine tumors. Clin Cancer Res 2000;6:2501–5.

Role for Radiation Therapy in Melanoma

Wenyin Shi, MD, PhD

KEYWORDS

- Radiation treatment • Stereotactic radiosurgery (SRS)
- Stereotactic body radiation treatment (SBRT) • Melanoma

KEY POINTS

- Definitive radiation plays an important role in early stage ocular melanoma with high local control and organ preservation.
- Definitive radiation therapy (RT) may be a viable option for lentigo maligna, lentigo maligna melanoma, and unresectable mocusal melanoma.
- Adjuvant RT following lymphadenectomy in node-positive melanoma prevents local and regional recurrence; however, it does not improve survival.
- Palliative radiation treatment is an important treatment option for metastatic melanoma, particularly with new stereotactic radiosurgery and stereotactic body radiotherapy techniques.
- A combination of radiation treatment and immunotherapy holds promise and is being actively evaluated.

INTRODUCTION

Radiation therapy (RT) works by damaging the DNA of cancer cells.
Radiation treatment techniques are divided into the following catagories.

External Beam Radiotherapy or Teletherapy

RT is delivered from a relatively distant source. The most common equipment is linear accelerators (LINAC). LINAC can produce both electron beams, suitable for superficial targets, and radiographic beams, suitable for deeper internal targets. The external beam radiotherapy (EBRT) radiation therapy treatment has been revolutionized with the advancement of computer software technology, high-resolution computed tomography (CT) and MRI imaging, and advanced delivery techniques.[1] It has evolved

The author received research funding for clinical trials from Bristol-Myers Squibb, Roche, Norvatis, and Millennium Pharmaceuticals.
Department of Radiation Oncology, Thomas Jefferson University, 111 South 11th Street, Suite G301, Philadelphia, PA 19107, USA
E-mail address: Wenyin.shi@jefferson.edu

Surg Oncol Clin N Am 24 (2015) 323–335
http://dx.doi.org/10.1016/j.soc.2014.12.009
1055-3207/15/$ – see front matter © 2015 Elsevier Inc. All rights reserved.

from 2-dimensional RT to 3-dimensional conformal RT, and currently, intensity-modulated RT, volumetric-modulated arc therapy as well as special techniques, such as stereotactic radiosurgery (SRS) and stereotactic body radiotherapy (SBRT) (**Fig. 1**).[2] Besides radiography (photon), proton radiation treatment is a special form of EBRT using charged particles. Protons penetrate tissue to a certain depth and deposit the energy in the tissue in a sharp peak, known as the Bragg peak. The Bragg peak of physical dose distribution permits the accurate concentration of the dose on the tumor, thus sparing the adjacent normal tissues.[3] It is particularly appealing for pediatric populations, and cancers close to critical structures, such as skull base, spine, and uveal melanoma.[4–8] Other particle radiation also has been used for clinical treatment, including neutron, and carbon ions.[6,9–11] However, their availability is very limited.

Brachytherapy

The radiation source is placed inside or next to the treatment area. Brachytherapy (BT) has the advantage of delivering high doses of radiation to the tumor while reducing the dose to the surrounding normal tissues. However, its use is greatly limited by the location and accessibility of the tumors.[12–14] Invasive procedures are needed for access to internal organ or deep target.

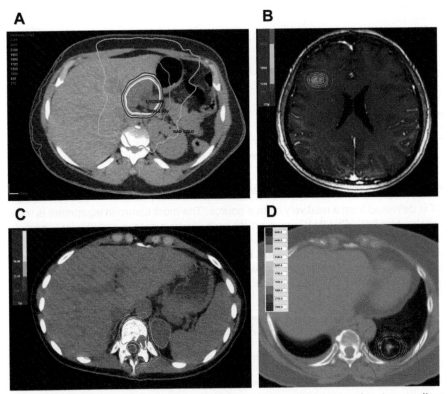

Fig. 1. Sample SRS and SBRT treatment plans for melanoma metastases, showing excellent radiation dose conformity and steep dose fall-off outside target. (*A*) SBRT for liver metastasis, (*B*) SRS for brain metastasis, (*C*) SRS for spine metastasis, (*D*) SBRT for lung metastasis.

Unsealed Source Radiotherapy

The soluble forms of radioactive substances are administered to the body by injection or ingestion. Examples are 131 iodine, 90 yttrium (90 Y) resin microsphere, and 223 radium dichloride.

Historically, melanoma is considered a relative radioresistant tumor. This notion primarily arose from cell culture studies, which showed a broad shoulder in the cell survival curves, suggesting a high repair capacity.[15–18] The high ability to repair DNA damage would make melanoma cells more sensitive to large RT dose per fraction.[19] Early clinical observations with large dose per fraction treatment resulted in conflicting results.[18,20,21] A multicenter randomized phase III trial (RTOG 83-05) attempted to address this question.[22] In this trial, 137 patients with measurable lesions were randomized to 2.5 Gy for 20 fractions and 8 Gy for 4 fractions. No difference in local control was observed. Unfortunately, the duration of response or survival was not reported. Retrospective studies comparing conventional and hypofractionated regimens in the adjuvant setting also failed to find significant differences.[23–26] On the other hand, a prospective randomized trial of different hypofractionated regimens (9 Gy × 3 vs 8 Gy × 5, 2 fractions per week) resulted in similar durable complete responses.[27] Taken together, the bias is to treat with the hypofractionated schedule with a fraction dose of 2.5 Gy or higher in the absence of contraindications. It is more convenient and generally well tolerated with a low risk of late complications.

Considering the treatment intent and relation with other modalities, the role of RT for melanoma can be divided into definitive treatment, adjuvant treatment, and palliative treatment.

DEFINITIVE RADIATION THERAPY FOR THE MELANOMA

Adequate surgery offers the best chance of local control and cure for primary melanoma. Definitive RT may be considered in certain special situations, such as inoperability due to medical comorbidities, location, or patient refusal.

Definitive Radiation Therapy for Lentigo Maligna and Lentigo Maligna Melanoma

Lentigo maligna (LM) and lentigo maligna melanoma (LMM) frequently affect elderly patients and may involve large areas of the face near critical structures.[28] Definitive RT has been used with good long-term local control with acceptable cosmetic and functional outcomes.[29–33] A pooled analysis of 349 patients with LM treated with definitive RT showed a 5% local recurrence rate. Salvage was successful in most of the recurrent LM by further RT, surgery, or other therapies.[34] A recent retrospective comparative study also revealed no statistical significant difference in outcome between surgery and RT for cutaneous melanoma.[35]

Definitive Radiation Therapy for Mucosal Melanoma

In a series of 28 patients with mucosal melanoma, actuarial local control of 49% was achieved at 3 years with 50 to 55 Gy in 15 to 16 fractions.[36] Similar local control of 44% was reported in 25 patients treated with 8 Gy delivered on days 0, 7, and 21.[37] A report on 31 patients from multiple institutes treated with definitive RT showed a local control of 58.1%. The authors concluded that hypofractionation with a dose per fraction greater than 3 Gy was associated with better local control and survival.[38] Taking into account some preliminary results with particle radiation, a pooled analysis showed local control as high as 70% can be achieved with RT alone.[39] Taken together, primary RT should be attempted for localized inoperable mucosal melanoma.

Definitive Radiation Therapy for Ocular Melanoma

Ocular melanoma is the most common primary intraocular malignant tumor in adults.[40] Successful treatment of ocular melanoma with eye and vision preservation is one of the major triumphs of radiation oncology. Very high rates of local control can be achieved with particle radiation treatment or episcleral plaque BT.[41]

Episcleral plaque brachytherapy for ocular melanoma

Initial experiences of episcleral BT used the high-energy isotope, 60 cobalt (60 Co).[42] Since then, low-energy isotopes, such as 125 iodine (125 I), 192 iridium, 131 cesium, 103 protactinium, and 106 ruthenium/106 rhodium, have replaced 60 Co.[43] 125 I is currently the most commonly used isotope. The Collaborative Ocular Melanoma Study conducted a 12-year study that demonstrated relative equivalence of 125 I plaque (85 Gy) compared with enucleation in the prevention of metastatic melanoma for medium-sized choroidal melanoma. Plaque BT was effective in sterilizing the gross tumor, with local control being achieved in approximately 90% of patients. However, radiation-induced ocular injury necessitated enucleation in approximately 5% of patients.[44] Retrospective analyses suggest lower doses can achieve similar rates of disease control with lower rates of toxicities.[45] Doses as low as 69 Gy may achieve similar rates of local control, distant metastasis-free survival, and overall survival as compared with 85 Gy.[45] To minimize the potential of visual acuity loss, for tumors close to macula, a dose less than 70 Gy to the tumor apex should be considered.[46]

Particle beam radiation therapy for ocular melanoma

Proton therapy is most commonly used for the treatment of ocular melanoma. It has the advantage over plaque therapy to treat larger tumors. For uveal melanoma, doses of 60 Gy delivered in 4 daily fractions of 15 Gy is highly effective.[47] Actuarial 15-year local control rate is 95%, and eye preservation rate is 84%, based on an analysis of 2069 patients treated at Harvard Cyclotron laboratory and Proton Therapy Center at Massachusetts General Hospital between 1975 and 1997.[47] A meta-analysis of 8809 patients with uveal melanoma included 7457 patients treated with charged particle therapy and 1352 patients with BT or enucleation. The rate of local recurrence was significantly lower with charged particle therapy than with BT (odds ratio 0.22). However, there were no significant differences in mortality or enucleation rates. Charged particle therapy was also associated with lower retinopathy and cataract formation rates.[6] A prospective randomized trial of lower-dose (50 Gy) versus standard-dose (70 Gy) proton radiation for small-size to moderate-size uveal melanoma showed no differences in 5-year local or systemic recurrence or visual acuity loss.[48]

ADJUVANT RADIATION THERAPY FOR MELANOMA

Adjuvant Radiation Therapy for Primary Melanoma

The mainstay of treatment of cutaneous melanoma is surgery. Adjuvant radiation treatment can be used to reduce the risk of local-regional failure in patients who are at high risk of recurrence; this is based on retrospective studies and has not been defined by clinical trials. The common factors of high risk of local-regional recurrence include close positive margins, lymphatic space invasion, multiple recurrences, desmoplastic or neurotropic growth, extensive satellitosis, and mucosal melanoma.[49–51] In these high-risk situations, adjuvant radiation treatment has a potential to reduce the risk of local-regional failure.[51–53] Desmoplastic neurotropic growth is an unusual subtype of melanoma and is reported to have a high local recurrence rate of 20% to 50% after surgery.[54] The benefit of adjuvant radiation is controversial.[54,55] Recent analysis showed only 8% of such patients in the United States received RT. As a result, the

North Central Cancer Center Treatment Group conducted a single-arm phase II trial to assess the role of adjuvant RT (NCT00060333). The result has not been reported yet. There is also a current randomized trial comparing adjuvant RT (48 Gy in 20 fractions) to observation for patients with primary melanoma of the head and neck region with neurotropism (NCT00975520). Results from these prospective studies would help define the role of adjuvant RT.

Adjuvant Radiation Therapy for Regional Lymphatic Metastases

Adjuvant radiation treatment after surgery decreases the rate of local recurrence for patients at high risk of regional failure after lymph node dissection; however, it does not improve overall survival. Risk factors for regional failure generally include multiple positive lymph nodes, large lymph node, extracapsular extension, and recurrence after prior lymph node dissection.[49,51,56–59] Some of the largest retrospective series are from MD Anderson Cancer Center. The RT regimen is 30 Gy in 5 fractions over a period of 2.5 weeks. Local control is 94% for head and neck melanoma, 87% for axilla, and 74% for ilioinguinal disease.[57–59] A prospective trial done in the 1970s was inconclusive.[60] It has several significant problems, including small sample size (56 patients total, 27 in the adjuvant RT arm, and 29 in the surgery alone arm), inadequate RT (50 Gy in 28 fractions), and short follow-up time. The most meaningful data are from the phase III trial by the Australia and New Zealand Melanoma Trials Group and Trans-Tasman Radiation Oncology Group.[61] Following surgery, 250 patients with positive lymph nodes deemed to be at high risk for locoregional recurrence were randomly assigned to RT (48 Gy in 20 fractions) or observation. Patients were considered at high risk if there was extracapsular extension, multiple positive nodes ($\geq$1 for parotid, $\geq$2 for neck and axilla, and $\geq$3 for groin location), and large lymph node ($\geq$3 cm for parotid, neck, and axilla, and $\geq$4 for groin location). After a median follow-up of 40 months, the radiation arm showed a significantly lower rate of lymph node recurrence as compared with observation. However, there were no differences in relapse-free survival or overall survival.[61] An update presented at American Society of Clinical Oncology 2013 meeting with 6-year median follow-up confirmed these findings. The 5-year local recurrence rate was 18% for the RT arm and 33% for the observation arm ($P = .02$), and no difference in relapse-free or overall survival.[62]

RADIATION THERAPY FOR DISTANT METASTASIS

RT is most commonly used for palliation for melanoma distant metastasis. Palliative treatments are for the relief of symptoms, and RT is effective for pain, mass effect, tumor-related hemorrhage, local irritation from skin, or subcutaneous lesions.[63] New RT techniques, such as SRS and SBRT, can achieve high probability of local control with very limited toxicity and are often preferred because of the relative radio-resistant nature of melanoma.

Brain metastases occur in more than 50% of patients with advanced melanoma.[64] The median survival of these patients is 4.4 months and the 5-year survival rate is approximately 3%.[65] Most of these patients die from central nervous system–related causes.[66] Surgery, whole brain radiation therapy (WBRT), and SRS are all used in the treatment of brain metastasis; nonetheless, the best treatment remains controversial and many patients receive more than one modality.[67,68] Radiation treatment is commonly used and effective. It results in symptomatic improvement and improved survival time.[69] Melanoma is considered a less radiosensitive tumor, and the local control with WBRT is poor. The estimated local control rates with WBRT at 6 and 12 months are 37% and 15%.[70] For patients with fewer metastases, SRS can be used as an alternative.[71–74] SRS treatment significantly improved the local control rate of melanoma brain metastases compared with those treated with WBRT.[75,76] The 12-month local control rate with SRS is about 65%.[73–76] Local control for other metastatic diseases, such as bone/spine, lung, and liver, treated with SRS/SBRT is also very favorable (70%–90%).[77–82] SBRT treatment also has the advantage of better pain control for bone metastasis. A large series of 500 patients (including melanoma) with spinal metastasis receiving single-fraction SRS treatment showed a long-term tumor control of 90%, and long-term pain control of 85%.[83]

Aggressive local treatment with SRS or SBRT to the sites of metastases may be particularly meaningful in a clinical significant disease state of oligometastases.[84] Multiple series indicate that 5-year survival can be as high as 15% to 41% in patients with a few sites of distant metastases that can be completely resected.[85–98] Ablative radiation treatment with SRS or SBRT can be a particularly useful alternative. The University of Rochester reported 2 protocols of patients with 1 to 5 metastases (mainly breast, lung, and colon primary) treated with SBRT.[99] The local control rate is 77% at 2 years. A similar experience from Duke University showed a 2-year local control rate of 52.7%,[100] warranting evaluation in patients with metastatic melanoma.

The liver is another common site for visceral melanoma metastasis and is involved in 15% to 20% of metastatic cutaneous melanoma,[101,102] and up to 95% of metastatic ocular melanoma.[103,104] Besides standard EBRT treatment, 90 Y radioembolization presents a new and attractive option for the management of liver metastasis. This radiation is a special form established for the treatment of hepatocellular carcinoma and liver metastasis.[105–107] Existing experiences suggest it is an effective and safe option for managing hepatic metastasis from melanoma (**Fig. 2**).[108–112] Further studies will help establish its role and optimal patient selection.

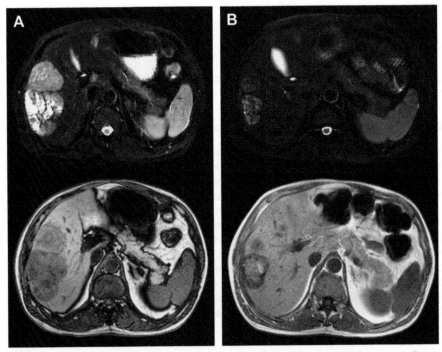

Fig. 2. A sample case of hepatic metastasis from uveal melanoma treated with 90 Y radioembolization. (*A*) Pretreatment MRI; (*B*) 3-m after-treatment MRI showed excellent response.

SUMMARY

RT clearly has a role in the management of melanoma. With the availability of new evidence, the practice pattern may continue to evolve. One of the key questions is how to best combine RT with systematic treatment. Combination of radiation with conventional chemotherapy may increase toxicity and thus generally is not used. Combining RT with immunotherapy may be very attractive for the management of melanoma. Treatment with RT would result in tumor cell death, releasing tumor debris and liberating potential tumor antigens. Previous reports support that RT modulates the immune system.[113,114] Initial experiences of combining radiation with interferon unfortunately showed significant toxicities.[115–117] However, RT may be of benefit and can be safely combined with newer immunotherapy agents, such as ipilimumab. Ipilimumab, a monoclonal antibody against cytotoxic T-lymphocyte antigen 4, was approved by the US Food and Drug Administration in 2011 for the treatment of unresectable and metastatic melanoma mainly based on the trials that showed improvement in overall survival.[118,119] Combining RT with ipilimumab may facilitate immune recognition of these novel tumor-specific antigens, focus the immune system on tumor antigens, and thus minimize the aberrant immune activation in normal tissues, consequently reducing the incidence of immune-related adverse effects. More importantly, a combination of radiation treatment with ipilimumab may also increase therapeutic effects. Clinical evidence has begun to accumulate for this combination.[114,120–122] Currently, the combination of ipilimumab and RT is being evaluated in more than 10 clinical trials (www.clinicaltrial.gov). In addition, several other immunomodulatory antibody approaches are also being developed at different stages, such as those to programmed death-1 and programmed death ligand-1.[123–125] Enthusiasm also exists for combining RT with molecular targeting approaches, such as BRAF inhibitors, Met inhibitors, Mek inhibitors.

Further advances of melanoma management will remain multidisciplinary approaches. Although the role of RT in the particular setting of melanoma management will continue to evolve, it is clear RT will remain one of the key therapeutic options in the multidisciplinary care for patients with melanoma.

REFERENCES

1. Bucci MK, Bevan A, Roach M. Advances in radiation therapy: conventional to 3D, to IMRT, to 4D, and beyond. CA Cancer J Clin 2005;55:117–34.
2. Noda SE, Lautenschlaeger T, Siedow MR, et al. Technological advances in radiation oncology for central nervous system tumors. Semin Radiat Oncol 2009;19: 179–86.
3. Jiang GL. Particle therapy for cancers: a new weapon in radiation therapy. Front Med 2012;6:165–72.
4. Munzenrider JE, Liebsch NJ. Proton therapy for tumors of the skull base. Strahlenther Onkol 1999;175(Suppl 2):57–63.
5. Munzenrider JE. Proton therapy for uveal melanomas and other eye lesions. Strahlenther Onkol 1999;175(Suppl 2):68–73.
6. Wang Z, Nabhan M, Schild SE, et al. Charged particle radiation therapy for uveal melanoma: a systematic review and meta-analysis. Int J Radiat Oncol Biol Phys 2013;86:18–26.
7. Merchant TE. Clinical controversies: proton therapy for pediatric tumors. Semin Radiat Oncol 2013;23:97–108.
8. Allen AM, Pawlicki T, Dong L, et al. An evidence based review of proton beam therapy: the report of ASTRO's emerging technology committee. Radiother Oncol 2012;103:8–11.

9. Laramore GE, Krall JM, Griffin TW, et al. Neutron versus photon irradiation for unresectable salivary gland tumors: final report of an RTOG-MRC randomized clinical trial. Radiation Therapy Oncology Group. Medical Research Council. Int J Radiat Oncol Biol Phys 1993;27:235–40.

10. Liao JJ, Parvathaneni U, Laramore GE, et al. Fast neutron radiotherapy for primary mucosal melanomas of the head and neck. Head Neck 2014;36: 1162–7.

11. Demizu Y, Fujii O, Terashima K, et al. Particle therapy for mucosal melanoma of the head and neck. A single-institution retrospective comparison of proton and carbon ion therapy. Strahlenther Onkol 2014;190:186–91.

12. Marwaha G, Macklis R, Singh AD, et al. Brachytherapy. Dev Ophthalmol 2013; 52:29–35.

13. McGuire SE, Frank SJ, Eifel PJ. Treatment of recurrent vaginal melanoma with external beam radiation therapy and palladium-103 brachytherapy. Brachytherapy 2008;7:359–63.

14. Krohn J, Dahl O, Nybø T, et al. Brachytherapy for malignant uveal melanoma. Tidsskr Nor Laegeforen 2014;134:529.

15. Barranco SC, Romsdahl MM, Humphrey RM. The radiation response of human malignant melanoma cells grown in vitro. Cancer Res 1971;31:830–3.

16. Dewey DL. The radiosensitivity of melanoma cells in culture. Br J Radiol 1971; 44:816–7.

17. Fertil B, Malaise EP. Intrinsic radiosensitivity of human cell lines is correlated with radioresponsiveness of human tumors: analysis of 101 published survival curves. Int J Radiat Oncol Biol Phys 1985;11:1699–707.

18. Rofstad EK. Radiation biology of malignant melanoma. Acta Radiol Oncol 1986; 25:1–10.

19. Jones B, Dale RG, Deehan C, et al. The role of biologically effective dose (BED) in clinical oncology. Clin Oncol (R Coll Radiol) 2001;13:71–81.

20. Bentzen SM, Overgaard J, Thames HD, et al. Clinical radiobiology of malignant melanoma. Radiother Oncol 1989;16:169–82.

21. Overgaard J. The role of radiotherapy in recurrent and metastatic malignant melanoma: a clinical radiobiological study. Int J Radiat Oncol Biol Phys 1986; 12:867–72.

22. Sause WT, Cooper JS, Rush S, et al. Fraction size in external beam radiation therapy in the treatment of melanoma. Int J Radiat Oncol Biol Phys 1991;20: 429–32.

23. Dvorák E, Haas RE, Liebner EJ. Contribution of radiotherapy to the management of malignant melanoma. A ten year experience at the University of Illinois Hospital in Chicago. Neoplasma 1993;40:387–99.

24. Fenig E, Eidelevich E, Njuguna E, et al. Role of radiation therapy in the management of cutaneous malignant melanoma. Am J Clin Oncol 1999;22:184–6.

25. Chang DT, Amdur RJ, Morris CG, et al. Adjuvant radiotherapy for cutaneous melanoma: comparing hypofractionation to conventional fractionation. Int J Radiat Oncol Biol Phys 2006;66:1051–5.

26. Strojan P, Jancar B, Cemazar M, et al. Melanoma metastases to the neck nodes: role of adjuvant irradiation. Int J Radiat Oncol Biol Phys 2010;77:1039–45.

27. Overgaard J, von der Maase H, Overgaard M. A randomized study comparing two high-dose per fraction radiation schedules in recurrent or metastatic malignant melanoma. Int J Radiat Oncol Biol Phys 1985;11:1837–9.

28. Weedon D. Melanoma and other melanocytic skin lesions. Curr Top Pathol 1985; 74:1–55.

29. De Groot WP. Provisional results of treatment of the mélanose précancéreuse circonscrite Dubreuilh by Bucky-rays. Dermatologica 1968;136:429–31.
30. Farshad A, Burg G, Panizzon R, et al. A retrospective study of 150 patients with lentigo maligna and lentigo maligna melanoma and the efficacy of radiotherapy using Grenz or soft X-rays. Br J Dermatol 2002;146:1042–6.
31. Panizzon R. Radiotherapy of lentigo maligna and lentigo maligna melanoma. Skin Cancer 1999;14:203–7.
32. Schmid-Wendtner MH, Brunner B, Konz B, et al. Fractionated radiotherapy of lentigo maligna and lentigo maligna melanoma in 64 patients. J Am Acad Dermatol 2000;43:477–82.
33. Hedblad MA, Mallbris L. Grenz ray treatment of lentigo maligna and early lentigo maligna melanoma. J Am Acad Dermatol 2012;67:60–8.
34. Fogarty GB, Hong A, Scolyer RA, et al. Radiotherapy for lentigo maligna: a literature review and recommendations for treatment. Br J Dermatol 2014;170:52–8.
35. Zalaudek I, Horn M, Richtig E, et al. Local recurrence in melanoma in situ: influence of sex, age, site of involvement and therapeutic modalities. Br J Dermatol 2003;148:703–8.
36. Gilligan D, Slevin NJ. Radical radiotherapy for 28 cases of mucosal melanoma in the nasal cavity and sinuses. Br J Radiol 1991;64:1147–50.
37. Harwood AR, Cummings BJ. Radiotherapy for mucosal melanomas. Int J Radiat Oncol Biol Phys 1982;8:1121–6.
38. Wada H, Nemoto K, Ogawa Y, et al. A multi-institutional retrospective analysis of external radiotherapy for mucosal melanoma of the head and neck in Northern Japan. Int J Radiat Oncol Biol Phys 2004;59:495–500.
39. Krengli M, Jereczek-Fossa BA, Kaanders JH, et al. What is the role of radiotherapy in the treatment of mucosal melanoma of the head and neck? Crit Rev Oncol Hematol 2008;65:121–8.
40. Siegel R, Naishadham D, Jemal A. Cancer statistics, 2013. CA Cancer J Clin 2013;63:11–30.
41. Munzenrider JE. Uveal melanomas. Conservation treatment. Hematol Oncol Clin North Am 2001;15:389–402.
42. Stallard HB. Radiotherapy for malignant melanoma of the choroid. Br J Ophthalmol 1966;50:147–55.
43. American Brachytherapy Society - Ophthalmic Oncology Task Force (ABS – OOTF) Committee. The American Brachytherapy Society consensus guidelines for plaque brachytherapy of uveal melanoma and retinoblastoma. Brachytherapy 2014;13:1–14.
44. Melia BM, Abramson DH, Albert DM, et al. Collaborative ocular melanoma study (COMS) randomized trial of I-125 brachytherapy for medium choroidal melanoma. I. Visual acuity after 3 years COMS report no. 16. Ophthalmology 2001;108:348–66.
45. Perez BA, Mettu P, Vajzovic L, et al. Uveal melanoma treated with iodine-125 episcleral plaque: an analysis of dose on disease control and visual outcomes. Int J Radiat Oncol Biol Phys 2014;89:127–36.
46. Jones R, Gore E, Mieler W, et al. Posttreatment visual acuity in patients treated with episcleral plaque therapy for choroidal melanomas: dose and dose rate effects. Int J Radiat Oncol Biol Phys 2002;52:989–95.
47. Gragoudas E, Li W, Goitein M, et al. Evidence-based estimates of outcome in patients irradiated for intraocular melanoma. Arch Ophthalmol 2002;120:1665–71.
48. Gragoudas ES, Lane AM, Regan S, et al. A randomized controlled trial of varying radiation doses in the treatment of choroidal melanoma. Arch Ophthalmol 2000;118:773–8.

49. Strojan P. Role of radiotherapy in melanoma management. Radiol Oncol 2010; 44:1–12.
50. Hong A, Fogarty G. Role of radiation therapy in cutaneous melanoma. Cancer J 2012;18:203–7.
51. Mendenhall WM, Shaw C, Amdur RJ, et al. Surgery and adjuvant radiotherapy for cutaneous melanoma considered high-risk for local-regional recurrence. Am J Otolaryngol 2013;34:320–2.
52. Cooper JS, Chang WS, Oratz R, et al. Elective radiation therapy for high-risk malignant melanomas. Cancer J 2001;7:498–502.
53. Ang KK, Peters LJ, Weber RS, et al. Postoperative radiotherapy for cutaneous melanoma of the head and neck region. Int J Radiat Oncol Biol Phys 1994;30: 795–8.
54. Guadagnolo BA, Prieto V, Weber R, et al. The role of adjuvant radiotherapy in the local management of desmoplastic melanoma. Cancer 2014;120:1361–8.
55. Wasif N, Gray RJ, Pockaj BA. Desmoplastic melanoma - the step-child in the melanoma family? J Surg Oncol 2011;103:158–62.
56. Agrawal S, Kane JM, Guadagnolo BA, et al. The benefits of adjuvant radiation therapy after therapeutic lymphadenectomy for clinically advanced, high-risk, lymph node-metastatic melanoma. Cancer 2009;115:5836–44.
57. Ballo MT, Bonnen MD, Garden AS, et al. Adjuvant irradiation for cervical lymph node metastases from melanoma. Cancer 2003;97:1789–96.
58. Ballo MT, Strom EA, Zagars GK, et al. Adjuvant irradiation for axillary metastases from malignant melanoma. Int J Radiat Oncol Biol Phys 2002;52:964–72.
59. Ballo MT, Zagars GK, Gershenwald JE, et al. A critical assessment of adjuvant radiotherapy for inguinal lymph node metastases from melanoma. Ann Surg Oncol 2004;11:1079–84.
60. Creagan ET, Cupps RE, Ivins JC, et al. Adjuvant radiation therapy for regional nodal metastases from malignant melanoma: a randomized, prospective study. Cancer 1978;42:2206–10.
61. Burmeister BH, Henderson MA, Ainslie J, et al. Adjuvant radiotherapy versus observation alone for patients at risk of lymph-node field relapse after therapeutic lymphadenectomy for melanoma: a randomised trial. Lancet Oncol 2012;13: 589–97.
62. Henderson M. Adjuvant radiotherapy after lymphadenectomy in melanoma patients: final results of an intergroup randomized trial (ANZMTG 1.02/TROG 02.01), ASCO annual meeting. Chicago, May 31 – June 4, 2013.
63. Fogarty GB, Hong A. Radiation therapy for advanced and metastatic melanoma. J Surg Oncol 2014;109:370–5.
64. Bafaloukos D, Gogas H. The treatment of brain metastases in melanoma patients. Cancer Treat Rev 2004;30:515–20.
65. Barth A, Wanek LA, Morton DL. Prognostic factors in 1,521 melanoma patients with distant metastases. J Am Coll Surg 1995;181:193–201.
66. Sampson JH, Carter JH Jr, Friedman AH, et al. Demographics, prognosis, and therapy in 702 patients with brain metastases from malignant melanoma. J Neurosurg 1998;88:11–20.
67. Andrews DW. Current neurosurgical management of brain metastases. Semin Oncol 2008;35:100–7.
68. Thomas SS, Dunbar EM. Modern multidisciplinary management of brain metastases. Curr Oncol Rep 2010;12:34–40.
69. Chu FC, Hilaris BB. Value of radiation therapy in the management of intracranial metastases. Cancer 1961;14:577–81.

70. Meyners T, Heisterkamp C, Kueter JD, et al. Prognostic factors for outcomes after whole-brain irradiation of brain metastases from relatively radioresistant tumors: a retrospective analysis. BMC Cancer 2010;10:582.

71. DiLuna ML, King JT Jr, Knisely JP, et al. Prognostic factors for survival after stereotactic radiosurgery vary with the number of cerebral metastases. Cancer 2007;109:135–45.

72. Manon R, O'Neill A, Knisely J, et al. Phase II trial of radiosurgery for one to three newly diagnosed brain metastases from renal cell carcinoma, melanoma, and sarcoma: an Eastern Cooperative Oncology Group study (E 6397). J Clin Oncol 2005;23:8870–6.

73. Mathieu D, Kondziolka D, Cooper PB, et al. Gamma knife radiosurgery for malignant melanoma brain metastases. Clin Neurosurg 2007;54:241–7.

74. Clarke JW, Register S, McGregor JM, et al. Stereotactic radiosurgery with or without whole brain radiotherapy for patients with a single radioresistant brain metastasis. Am J Clin Oncol 2010;33:70–4.

75. Powell JW, Chung CT, Shah HR, et al. Gamma Knife surgery in the management of radioresistant brain metastases in high-risk patients with melanoma, renal cell carcinoma, and sarcoma. J Neurosurg 2008;109(Suppl):122–8.

76. Lo SS, Clarke JW, Grecula JC, et al. Stereotactic radiosurgery alone for patients with 1-4 radioresistant brain metastases. Med Oncol 2010;28(Suppl 1):S439–44.

77. Rule W, Timmerman R, Tong L, et al. Phase I dose-escalation study of stereotactic body radiotherapy in patients with hepatic metastases. Ann Surg Oncol 2011;18:1081–7.

78. Lo SS, Teh BS, Mayr NA, et al. Stereotactic body radiation therapy for oligometastases. Discov Med 2010;10:247–54.

79. Timmerman R, Paulus R, Galvin J, et al. Stereotactic body radiation therapy for inoperable early stage lung cancer. JAMA 2010;303:1070–6.

80. Rusthoven KE, Kavanagh BD, Cardenes H, et al. Multi-institutional phase I/II trial of stereotactic body radiation therapy for liver metastases. J Clin Oncol 2009;27:1572–8.

81. Hoyer M, Roed H, Traberg Hansen A, et al. Phase II study on stereotactic body radiotherapy of colorectal metastases. Acta Oncol 2006;45:823–30.

82. Chawla S, Chen Y, Katz AW, et al. Stereotactic body radiotherapy for treatment of adrenal metastases. Int J Radiat Oncol Biol Phys 2009;75:71–5.

83. Gerszten PC, Burton SA, Ozhasoglu C, et al. Radiosurgery for spinal metastases: clinical experience in 500 cases from a single institution. Spine (Phila Pa 1976) 2007;32:193–9.

84. Hellman S, Weichselbaum RR. Oligometastases. J Clin Oncol 1995;13:8–10.

85. Sosman JA, Moon J, Tuthill RJ, et al. A phase 2 trial of complete resection for stage IV melanoma: results of Southwest Oncology Group Clinical Trial S9430. Cancer 2011;117(20). 4740–06.

86. Ricaniadis N, Konstadoulakis MM, Walsh D, et al. Gastrointestinal metastases from malignant melanoma. Surg Oncol 1995;4:105–10.

87. Ollila DW, Essner R, Wanek LA, et al. Surgical resection for melanoma metastatic to the gastrointestinal tract. Arch Surg 1996;131:975–9, 979–80.

88. Agrawal S, Yao TJ, Coit DG. Surgery for melanoma metastatic to the gastrointestinal tract. Ann Surg Oncol 1999;6:336–44.

89. Harpole DH Jr, Johnson CM, Wolfe WG, et al. Analysis of 945 cases of pulmonary metastatic melanoma. J Thorac Cardiovasc Surg 1992;103:743–8 [discussion: 748–50].

90. Leo F, Cagini L, Rocmans P, et al. Lung metastases from melanoma: when is surgical treatment warranted? Br J Cancer 2000;83:569–72.
91. Tafra L, Dale PS, Wanek LA, et al. Resection and adjuvant immunotherapy for melanoma metastatic to the lung and thorax. J Thorac Cardiovasc Surg 1995; 110:119–28 [discussion: 129].
92. Ollila DW, Stern SL, Morton DL. Tumor doubling time: a selection factor for pulmonary resection of metastatic melanoma. J Surg Oncol 1998;69:206–11.
93. Karakousis CP, Velez A, Driscoll DL, et al. Metastasectomy in malignant melanoma. Surgery 1994;115:295–302.
94. Wong JH, Skinner KA, Kim KA, et al. The role of surgery in the treatment of nonregionally recurrent melanoma. Surgery 1993;113:389–94.
95. Fletcher WS, Pommier RF, Lum S, et al. Surgical treatment of metastatic melanoma. Am J Surg 1998;175:413–7.
96. Ollila DW, Hsueh EC, Stern SL, et al. Metastasectomy for recurrent stage IV melanoma. J Surg Oncol 1999;71:209–13.
97. Meyer T, Merkel S, Goehl J, et al. Surgical therapy for distant metastases of malignant melanoma. Cancer 2000;89:1983–91.
98. Ollila DW. Complete metastasectomy in patients with stage IV metastatic melanoma. Lancet Oncol 2006;7:919–24.
99. Milano MT, Katz AW, Muhs AG, et al. A prospective pilot study of curative-intent stereotactic body radiation therapy in patients with 5 or fewer oligometastatic lesions. Cancer 2008;112:650–8.
100. Salama JK, Hasselle MD, Chmura SJ, et al. Stereotactic body radiotherapy for multisite extracranial oligometastases: final report of a dose escalation trial in patients with 1 to 5 sites of metastatic disease. Cancer 2011;118(11):2962–70.
101. Leiter U, Meier F, Schittek B, et al. The natural course of cutaneous melanoma. J Surg Oncol 2004;86:172–8.
102. Cohn-Cedermark G, Månsson-Brahme E, Rutqvist LE, et al. Metastatic patterns, clinical outcome, and malignant phenotype in malignant cutaneous melanoma. Acta Oncol 1999;38:549–57.
103. Becker JC, Terheyden P, Kämpgen E, et al. Treatment of disseminated ocular melanoma with sequential fotemustine, interferon alpha, and interleukin 2. Br J Cancer 2002;87:840–5.
104. Trout AT, Rabinowitz RS, Platt JF, et al. Melanoma metastases in the abdomen and pelvis: frequency and patterns of spread. World J Radiol 2013;5:25–32.
105. Kennedy A. Radioembolization of hepatic tumors. J Gastrointest Oncol 2014;5: 178–89.
106. Memon K, Lewandowski RJ, Mulcahy MF, et al. Radioembolization for neuroendocrine liver metastases: safety, imaging, and long-term outcomes. Int J Radiat Oncol Biol Phys 2012;83:887–94.
107. Dezarn WA, Cessna JT, DeWerd LA, et al. Recommendations of the American Association of Physicists in Medicine on dosimetry, imaging, and quality assurance procedures for 90Y microsphere brachytherapy in the treatment of hepatic malignancies. Med Phys 2011;38:4824–45.
108. Xing M, Prajapati HJ, Dhanasekaran R, et al. Selective internal yttrium-90 radioembolization therapy (90Y-SIRT) versus best supportive care in patients with unresectable metastatic melanoma to the liver refractory to systemic therapy: safety and efficacy cohort study. Am J Clin Oncol 2014. [Epub ahead of print].
109. Memon K, Kuzel TM, Vouche M, et al. Hepatic yttrium-90 radioembolization for metastatic melanoma: a single-center experience. Melanoma Res 2014;24: 244–51.

110. Eldredge-Hindy H, Ohri N, Anne PR, et al. Yttrium-90 microsphere brachyther-apy for liver metastases from uveal melanoma: clinical outcomes and the pre-dictive value of fluorodeoxyglucose positron emission tomography. Am J Clin Oncol 2014. [Epub ahead of print].
111. Piduru SM, Schuster DM, Barron BJ, et al. Prognostic value of 18f-fluorodeoxy-glucose positron emission tomography-computed tomography in predicting sur-vival in patients with unresectable metastatic melanoma to the liver undergoing yttrium-90 radioembolization. J Vasc Interv Radiol 2012;23:943–8.
112. Klingenstein A, Haug AR, Zech CJ, et al. Radioembolization as locoregional therapy of hepatic metastases in uveal melanoma patients. Cardiovasc Intervent Radiol 2013;36:158–65.
113. Demaria S, Ng B, Devitt ML, et al. Ionizing radiation inhibition of distant un-treated tumors (abscopal effect) is immune mediated. Int J Radiat Oncol Biol Phys 2004;58:862–70.
114. Postow MA, Callahan MK, Barker CA, et al. Immunologic correlates of the ab-scopal effect in a patient with melanoma. N Engl J Med 2012;366:925–31.
115. Gyorki DE, Ainslie J, Joon ML, et al. Concurrent adjuvant radiotherapy and interferon-alpha2b for resected high risk stage III melanoma – a retrospective single centre study. Melanoma Res 2004;14:223–30.
116. Nguyen NP, Levinson B, Dutta S, et al. Concurrent interferon-alpha and radiation for head and neck melanoma. Melanoma Res 2003;13:67–71.
117. Conill C, Jorcano S, Domingo-Domènech J, et al. Toxicity of combined treatment of adjuvant irradiation and interferon alpha2b in high-risk melanoma patients. Melanoma Res 2007;17:304–9.
118. Hodi FS, O'Day SJ, McDermott DF, et al. Improved survival with ipilimumab in patients with metastatic melanoma. N Engl J Med 2010;363:711–23.
119. Robert C, Thomas L, Bondarenko I, et al. Ipilimumab plus dacarbazine for pre-viously untreated metastatic melanoma. N Engl J Med 2011;364:2517–26.
120. Knisely JP, Yu JB, Flanigan J, et al. Radiosurgery for melanoma brain metasta-ses in the ipilimumab era and the possibility of longer survival. J Neurosurg 2012;117:227–33.
121. Mathew M, Tam M, Ott PA, et al. Ipilimumab in melanoma with limited brain me-tastases treated with stereotactic radiosurgery. Melanoma Res 2013;23:191–5.
122. Bot I, Blank CU, Brandsma D. Clinical and radiological response of leptomenin-geal melanoma after whole brain radiotherapy and ipilimumab. J Neurol 2012; 259:1976–8.
123. Topalian SL, Sznol M, McDermott DF, et al. Survival, durable tumor remission, and long-term safety in patients with advanced melanoma receiving nivolumab. J Clin Oncol 2014;32:1020–30.
124. Topalian SL, Hodi FS, Brahmer JR, et al. Safety, activity, and immune correlates of anti-PD-1 antibody in cancer. N Engl J Med 2012;366:2443–54.
125. Hamid O, Robert C, Daud A, et al. Safety and tumor responses with lambrolizu-mab (anti-PD-1) in melanoma. N Engl J Med 2013;369:134–44.

Update on Immunotherapy in Melanoma

Jamie Green, MD, Charlotte Ariyan, MD, PhD*

KEYWORDS

- Immunotherapy • Antitumor immunity • Metastatic melanoma
- Costimulatory blockade • Innate immunity • Adaptive immunity

KEY POINTS

- Immunotherapy agents have been demonstrated to improve survival option for patients with metastatic melanoma.
- The field of immunotherapy now offers treatments with the potential for a long-term cure.
- As the field moves forward, studies will focus on improving the response rates with new immunotherapy agents or novel treatment combinations.

HISTORY OF IMMUNOTHERAPY

The idea of enhancing the immune response to reduce cancer growth can be traced back to Dr William Coley's work at New York Cancer Hospital more than a century ago. Dr Coley initially noted tumor regression in a patient who developed a postoperative infection. The patient had recurrent cheek sarcoma, underwent a partial excision of his tumor, and was cured of the remaining tumor after he developed a wound infection with the bacteria *Streptococcal pyogenes*.[1] Coley concluded that the immune response to the bacteria played an integral role in fighting the cancer. He then inoculated with bacteria his next 10 patients who had tumors that could not be surgically excised successfully. This approach had several problems, given that he saw a range of responses; some patients failed to develop an infection, whereas others developed too strong of an infection that it proved fatal. However, he did find that the patients who had an immune reaction to the bacteria, including fever and inflammation, experienced tumor reduction.[1] He subsequently tested the effect of injecting a vaccine with killed bacteria into the tumors, otherwise known as *Coley's toxin*, to stimulate an immune response without risking fatal infection, and found that he was able to cause complete regression of cancer in some patients.[1] Unfortunately, much of this work

The authors have nothing to declare.

Memorial Sloan Kettering Cancer Center, Department of Surgery, 1275 York Avenue, New York, NY 10065, USA

* Corresponding author.

E-mail address: ariyanc@mskcc.org

Surg Oncol Clin N Am 24 (2015) 337–346

http://dx.doi.org/10.1016/j.soc.2014.12.010

1055-3207/15/$ – see front matter

was abandoned for years after his death as a result of the discovery of radiation and cytotoxic chemotherapy.

However, over the past few decades, the field of immunotherapy has been reborn. Careful preclinical studies have enhanced the understanding of the immune system and ways to promote antitumor immunity, most specifically with the use of adoptive T cells, which are specific for the cancer itself, and immune checkpoint blockade. Prospective randomized trials have demonstrated the efficacy of immune checkpoint blockade in the treatment of melanoma, and the field continues to move forward at a rapid pace. Together these treatments have resulted in a cure for many patients and have changed the way in which metastatic melanoma is treated. This article focuses on the immune system, immunotherapy treatments for melanoma, and the new treatments in development that show potential for improved success.

THE IMMUNE SYSTEM

The human immune system comprises 2 main branches, innate and adaptive immunity, which work together to form a fast and effective response to a pathogen. Innate immunity involves nonspecific mechanisms to fight all foreign invaders. These cells are normally the first responders to an insult because they are always present in individuals and do not need time to develop. The first components of the innate immune response are anatomic barriers, such as the skin, which serves as a barrier to prevent the entry of microbes, and mucous membranes, which trap foreign organisms to remove them from the body; and physiologic barriers, such as the low pH of the stomach, which kills most organisms that are ingested.[2] The main cells involved in the innate immune response are (1) mast cells, which cause blood vessel dilation to increase flow to the injured area, and the release of chemokines, proteins that attract other immune cells to the area; (2) macrophages, which are large cells that phagocytose (engulf and digest) the bacteria and secrete immunostimulatory proteins, also referred to as *cytokines*; (3) neutrophils, which are the most abundant circulating white blood cell (WBC), and phagocytose bacteria or dead cells; (4) basophils and eosinophils, which secrete immunostimulatory proteins; and (5) natural killer cells, which destroy damaged or abnormal cells, including tumor cells, and are recognized by their lack of certain proteins, called *major histocompatibility complex* (MHC) class I, which are on the surface of all normal cells.[2]

On the other hand, the adaptive immune system generates a highly specific response, which depends on the exact pathogen that has invaded. It takes several days after the initial exposure to generate a notable response. Adaptive immunity exhibits memory and, on subsequent exposures to the same antigen, is able to generate a faster and stronger response.[2] The main cells of the adaptive immune response are B and T cells. Each B cell recognizes and binds to a specific antigen, causing the B cell to replicate and differentiate into plasma cells, which secrete antibodies specific for the antigen that then circulate in the blood and bind to the pathogen, leading to its elimination.

There are multiple types of T cells, including helper T cells, cytotoxic T cells, and regulatory T cells (Treg). In general, T cells require an interaction with other cells, called antigen-presenting cells (APCs), to be activated. When activated with antigen, an APC will bind to a T cell with a receptor (TCR) specific for that APC-antigen complex, providing the initial T cell stimulatory signal, or "signal one." For T cells to be fully activated, a second costimulatory signal is required, which is also known as "signal two." The best-characterized costimulatory interaction is between CD80 or CD86 on APC and CD28 on the surface of T cells. Once both signals occur simultaneously, the T cell is able to respond, secrete factors that activate other T cells, and differentiate into the different types of T cells.[2] Helper T cells secrete proteins that activate other immune cells, including B cells, cytotoxic T cells, and macrophages. Cytotoxic T cells are able to kill damaged or infected cells and cancer cells. Treg cells are a subset of lymphocytes that have a role in attenuating the immune response to help prevent excessive immune activation, and alterations in these cells are important in the pathogenesis of cancers and autoimmune conditions.[2]

IMMUNOTHERAPY AND MELANOMA

Melanoma is a highly aggressive cancer that is resistant to most available chemotherapy agents. An estimated 76,000 new cases of melanoma were diagnosed in the United States in 2014, with more than 9700 melanoma-related deaths. Although melanoma accounts for less than 5% of all skin cancers, it is responsible for 75% of skin cancer deaths.[3] The median survival for patients diagnosed with metastatic melanoma historically is only 6 to 9 months.[3] However, in the past few years, several exciting new therapies have been shown to improve overall survival.

Localized Bacillus Calmette-Guerin Injection

As noted, the field of immunotherapy has origins from the end of the 19th century (**Fig. 1**). The resurgence of the field was initiated in part through the hard work of Dr Lloyd Old who, among many things, established the importance of Bacillus Calmette-Guérin (BCG), tumor necrosis factor (TNF), and described numerous tumor to antigens. BCG, a live *Mycobacterium bovis* vaccine, was initially created in an attempt at generating a tuberculosis vaccine, but it was also found to have antitumor properties.[4] It was the first immunotherapy agent approved by the US Food and Drug Administration (FDA) for cancer treatment. Locally injected BCG is currently an effective treatment for early-stage bladder cancer, and BCG has also been studied in the treatment of melanoma, pioneered in part by Dr Donald Morton.[5] Intratumoral BCG injection for melanoma was associated with high response rates for localized disease, although this was not proven to be statistically significant and was associated with unacceptable toxicity.[6] BCG was also used in the randomized phase III study of the failed Canvaxin whole-cell vaccine in which patients were randomized to receive postoperative Canvaxin plus BCG or BCG plus placebo after tumor resection. Although the trial was discontinued because of failure to show a survival benefit with Canvaxin treatment, the higher survival seen in both arms of this trial when compared with similar

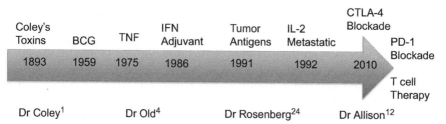

Immunotherapy Timeline

Coley's Toxins	BCG	TNF	IFN Adjuvant	Tumor Antigens	IL-2 Metastatic	CTLA-4 Blockade
1893	1959	1975	1986	1991	1992	2010

PD-1 Blockade

T cell Therapy

Dr Coley[1]   Dr Old[4]   Dr Rosenberg[24]   Dr Allison[12]

Fig. 1. The development of the field of immunotherapy has taken place over more than a century, with several key figures making novel discoveries to advance the field. IFN, interferon; PD-1, programmed death-1 receptor.

patients in other studies resulted in a renewed interest in BCG as a biological agent.[7] Recently, reduced doses of BCG in combination with other treatments, such as topical imiquimod, have demonstrated efficacy in small studies, although larger, randomized trials are still needed to evaluate the potential survival benefits of intratumoral BCG injection.[8]

Interleukin-2

Interleukin-2 (IL-2) was approved by the FDA for the treatment of malignant melanoma in 1998. IL-2, or T-cell growth factor, is normally secreted by T cells after the binding of antigen to the TCR, resulting in stimulation and increased activity of all types of T cells.[9] Early melanoma studies showed promising results with high-dose IL-2 treatment, resulting in the possibility of a long-term response in some patients. Unfortunately, few patients experience response to the treatment, with an overall response rate of 16% and a complete response, resulting in disappearance of all lesions, seen in only 6% of patients.[10] Additionally, no randomized controlled studies have shown a survival benefit with IL-2 treatment compared with standard chemotherapy regimens. Furthermore, IL-2 treatment is associated with a variety of adverse events, most of which are related to increased permeability of blood vessels, resulting in low blood pressure, elevated heart rate, and extremity swelling. Other side effects include rash, fever, nausea, vomiting, diarrhea, and infection.[11] These side effects can be managed well through adjusting the dose and administering the medication in an environment where experienced personnel can manage the side effects. However, the newer immunotherapy medications can be administered in the outpatient setting, and have shown improved efficacy in prospective randomized trials, and thus are replacing the use of IL-2 as a first-line treatment.

Immune Checkpoint Blockade

The field of immunotherapy was changed in 2011 when the FDA approved the first immune checkpoint inhibitor, ipilimumab (or Yervoy). Ipilimumab is a humanized antibody that binds to cytotoxic T-lymphocyte antigen 4 (CTLA-4) and blocks its activity. CTLA-4 is normally expressed on the surface of T cells after activation, and functions to turn off the T-cell response to prevent an excessive immune reaction. CTLA-4 binds to CD80 or CD86 on APC with a stronger bond than to CD28, displacing the costimulatory interaction and delivering a powerful negative signal to the TCR (**Fig. 2**). Dr James Allison[12] hypothesized that blocking this negative regulatory signal with an antibody would allow the immune response to continue and result in antitumor immunity. His preclinical work demonstrating efficacy in murine models was then moved forward into clinical trials.[12] Studies have demonstrated that anti–CTLA-4 treatments augment tumor-specific immunity through increasing the CD8/Treg ratio in the tumor and by directly depleting Treg cells through an Fcγ receptor–dependent mechanism, resulting in a rapid loss of these inhibitory cells from the tumor environment.[13,14]

The efficacy of CTLA-4 blockade was demonstrated in 2 prospective randomized control trials. The first trial involved 676 patients with stage III or IV melanoma who experienced disease progression while receiving an alternate form of systemic therapy (eg, chemotherapy and/or IL-2).[15] In this study, patients were randomized to receive ipilimumab alone, ipilimumab and a vaccine against a component of melanoma cells (called gp100), or gp100 alone. Patients who received ipilimumab, with or without gp100, showed a significant improvement in median survival (10.0 vs 6.4 months). No difference in survival was seen in patients who received gp100 with ipilimumab compared with those who received ipilimumab alone, showing no benefit

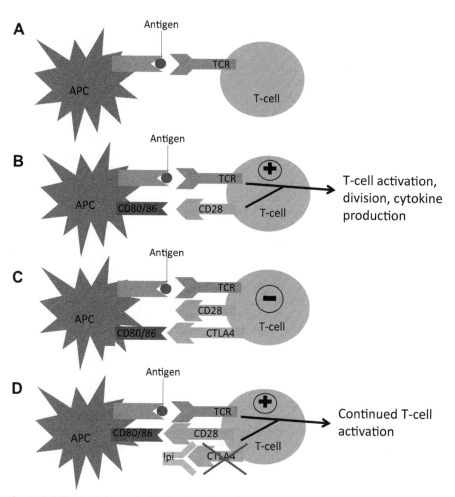

Fig. 2. (A) The initial step in T-cell activation is binding of the TCR to the antigen complex on the APC. (B) A second costimulatory interaction is required for activation, between CD80 or CD86 on APC and CD28 on the T cell. Once both interactions occur simultaneously, the T cell is activated, divides, and produces cytokines. (C) After activation, CTLA-4 is expressed on the surface, which has a stronger binding affinity to CD80 and CD86 and thus displaces CD28, turning off the T cell. (D) Ipilimumab (Ipi) binds to CTLA-4 so that it is unable to bind to CD80 or CD86, allowing a continued interaction with CD28 and continued T-cell activation.

to the vaccine. Unfortunately, as with IL-2 treatment, response rate to ipilimumab was low, with 10.9% of patients experiencing a partial or complete response and an additional 17.6% of patients showing stable disease. Sixty percent of responding patients had a continued response after 2 years.[15] Furthermore, long-term follow-up of patients from the phase III trial mentioned previously, and earlier phase I and II trials, have demonstrated the possibility of long-term survival (with some patients alive 10 years posttreatment), again highlighting the durability of the treatment responses.[16,17]

This landmark immunotherapy trial was confirmed by a second trial that compared ipilimumab plus dacarbazine, the only chemotherapy agent FDA-approved for melanoma treatment, versus dacarbazine plus placebo in 502 previously untreated patients with stage III or IV melanoma.[18] Again, in patients treated with ipilimumab, median overall survival was significantly increased (11.2 vs 9.1 months) and higher survival rates were seen at 1 year (47.4% vs 36.3%), 2 years (28.5% vs 17.9%), and 3 years (20.8% vs 12.2%). Similarly, the overall response rate in patients treated with ipilimumab was 15.2%. It is notable that the liver toxicity associated with combination treatment in this trial was higher than what had been noted with either treatment alone. Given that ipilimumab functions to increase immune system activation, it is not surprising that most adverse events in both studies were immune-related, including colitis, dermatitis, hepatitis, endocrinopathy, and neuritis. In contrast to autoimmune diseases, these toxicities can usually be managed with cessation of the drug and/or corticosteroid administration.[18]

The kinetics of response associated with ipilimumab treatment have been noted to differ greatly from those associated with other types of treatment, such as chemotherapy agents. Patients who receive ipilimumab may have a delayed response, which does not appear until more than 12 weeks posttreatment. This finding is thought to be related to the delay in effect seen with the normal adaptive immune response. With the immunomodulating agents, unlike with conventional chemotherapy agents, time is needed to activate the T cells, release stimulating proteins, recruit additional immune cells to the tumor site, and, finally, for the immune cells to destroy the tumor. Therefore, a new model was created to evaluate response to the immunotherapy drugs, called the *new immune-related response criteria*, to avoid overlooking patients that exhibit a delayed response.[19]

Given the results found with ipilimumab treatment, inhibition of alternate immune checkpoint proteins is currently being investigated. The other most extensively studied interaction is between programmed death-1 receptor (PD-1) on the surface of activated T cells with its ligand (PD-L1) on APC or tumor cells. PD-1, like CTLA-4, is expressed on the surface of activated T cells, as well as on "exhausted" T cells that have been exposed to overwhelming amounts of antigen and are no longer active.[20] When PD-1 binds PD-L1, it attenuates the immune response. The expression of PD-L1 on tumor cells is thought to play a role in decreased immune response in the tumor microenvironment, contributing to tumor growth and spread. Early studies of PD-1 and PD-L1 inhibition showed promising results in patients with melanoma. A phase I study[20] examined the safety of BMS-936558, a human monoclonal blocking antibody against PD-1, in 296 patients with advanced solid tumors, including melanoma, non–small cell lung cancer, prostate cancer, renal cell carcinoma, and colorectal cancer, for whom other treatment modalities failed (excluding anti–CTLA-4 or other PD-1/L1 agents). The toxicity profile was acceptable, and promising response rates were seen in patients with melanoma, non–small cell lung cancer, and renal cell cancer. For patients with advanced melanoma, the partial or complete response rate was 28% among all doses, and 41% at the highest dose (3.0 mg/kg), with 72% of patients who were followed for at least a year having long-term responses lasting more than a year. A similar study[21] was performed for BMS-936559, a human monoclonal antibody to PD-L1, that showed that the treatment was safe and that 17% of patients with melanoma experienced partial or complete responses to treatment. Randomized controlled trials evaluating survival benefits for PD-1 and PD-L1 inhibitors are currently being performed. Like ipilimumab, anti–PD-1/L1 medications have mostly immune-related adverse events.

Given the success of inhibiting these 2 isolated immunosuppressive interactions, early studies have been reported that are examining the combination of anti–CTLA-4 and anti–PD-1 medications. In a study published in the *New England Journal of Medicine* in 2013,[22] patients with metastatic melanoma who were naïve to T-cell–modulating agents were treated with concurrent nivolumab (anti-PD-1 antibody) and ipilimumab every 3 weeks for 4 doses followed by nivolumab alone every 3 weeks for 4 doses, and those who previously received at least 3 doses of ipilimumab who did not experience complete response or progression of disease were treated with nivolumab every 2 weeks. Adverse event rates were higher in patients receiving combination therapy than in those receiving the drugs separately; however, most adverse events were reversible. An impressive response rate of 40% was seen in patients receiving the concurrent dosing versus 20% in those treated with the sequenced regimen. A subsequent update[23] on this trial demonstrated an 82% survival rate at 1 year for the concurrent regimen and a 75% survival rate at 2 years. These exciting results show improved response rates with the combination of multiple immunotherapy agents, and suggest that patients who experience disease progression on one agent may still be able to benefit from the alternate agent. Given the results of these studies, as well as additional trials, nivolumab was approved by the FDA in December 2014 for the treatment of advanced melanoma after the failure of other treatments. The field is anxiously awaiting the results of current randomized controlled studies that are further evaluating the potential survival benefits of nivolumab and combination immunotherapy.

Adoptive T-Cell Transfer

Adoptive T-cell transfer, pioneered by Dr Steve Rosenberg,[24] is the concept of isolating T cells from a patient, expanding them in the laboratory, and then infusing them back into the patient with a goal of targeting the tumor with an increased strength than the body is naturally able to provide (**Fig. 3**). For solid tumors, this is usually performed using tumor-infiltrating lymphocytes (TILs) isolated from an excised tumor. A phase II trial of adoptive transfer of TILs in patients with stage IV melanoma published in 2010 showed an objective response in 50% of patients.[25] However, some patients are not eligible for this type of treatment because (1) they do not have a lesion that can be resected, (2) the resected tumor does not have any TILs that grow or demonstrate antitumor reactivity in vitro, (3) the patient's pace of disease is too quick to allow time for the ex vivo events to happen, or (4) the patient's medical condition is not strong enough to support the preinfusion conditioning regimen, which often involves cytotoxic chemotherapy and total body radiation.[24]

Chimeric antigen receptors (CARs) were introduced as a method of genetically modifying a patient's T cells to make them target tumor cells, without requiring tumor resection and TILs. CARs are molecules engineered onto T cells derived from the patient's blood that involve (1) an antigen-recognition domain that is able to recognize a specific protein on the surface of tumor cells, (2) a transmembrane portion, and (3) an intracellular domain that works similarly to the T cell receptor (TCR) to activate the T cell and stimulate in vivo proliferation.[26] Although most of the success thus far in CAR therapy has been in liquid tumors, with anti-CD19 CARs for the treatment of chronic lymphocytic leukemia leading the field, CAR therapy is also evolving in the treatment of melanoma.[27] A phase II study published in 2009 treated 36 patients with CAR therapy targeting melanocytic proteins overexpressed in melanoma (DMF5 or gp100). Although objective response rates of 30% and 19% were found for DMF5 and gp100 CARs, respectively, patients unfortunately also exhibited destruction of normal melanocytes, resulting in vitiligo, uveitis, and hearing loss.[28] Therefore, further studies and additional antigen targets for melanoma are needed. Although currently no FDA-approved adoptive T-cell therapies are available, numerous clinical trials

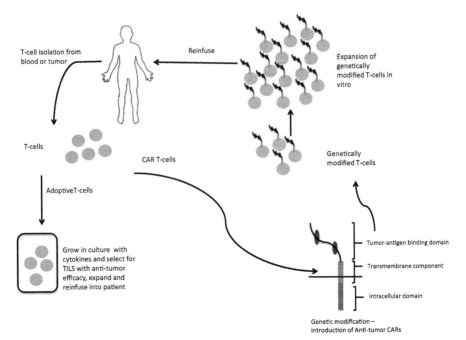

Fig. 3. Adoptive T-cell transfer. T cells are isolated from the tumor or blood of the patient. TILs isolated from the tumor are expanded in vitro then reinfused into the patient. Alternatively, T cells isolated from the patient's blood are genetically modified by adding a chimeric antigen receptor (CAR), which is specific for an antigen typically found on the tumor type being targeted. The genetically modified T cells are then expanded *in vitro* using T-cell growth factors and then reinfused into the patient to target the tumor.

are underway to determine their safety profiles on a larger scale and their effects on survival for numerous types of cancer.

FUTURE DIRECTIONS

The immunotherapy arena has exploded with the recent advances in melanoma, demonstrating an improvement in survival and, most importantly, a durability of response. The field is now investigating the role of new immunotherapies alone and in combination, such as (1) blockade of lymphocyte activation gene 3 (LAG3), which normally stimulates Treg cells and inhibits CD8+ effector T cells through its interaction with MHC class II molecules; (2) T-cell membrane protein 3 (Tim 3) antagonists, which have been shown to increase antitumor T-cell responses when used in combination with anti-PD1 agents; (3) B7-H3 blockade, which has been found to increase antitumor immunity in preclinical models; and (4) agonists of TNF receptor superfamily members 4-1BB, OX40, and GITR, which result in CD4+ and CD8+ T-cell activation.[29–32] Additional treatment combinations are also being investigated, such as combining immunotherapy with targeted therapy, for example BRAF inhibitors. Given the adverse event profiles of these medications, it is extremely important to investigate the new therapies carefully. Although blockade of negative signals has brought great success, treatment with agonists has been more difficult. For example, potentiation of a positive signal with a CD28 agonist resulted in a severe cytokine storm, and early studies of treatment with a 4-1BB agonist resulted in fatal hepatotoxicity.[33,34] These studies highlight the importance of careful preclinical work and clinical studies moving forward.

SUMMARY

Immunotherapy is now recognized as a viable option for patients with metastatic melanoma. Although this field has taken more than a century to mature, it now offers treatments with the potential for long-term cure. As the field moves forward, studies will focus on improving the response rates with new immunotherapy agents or novel treatment combinations. Given these promising preliminary results and the large number of trials currently underway, it is exciting to anticipate what the future will hold for the field of immunotherapy and the treatment of malignant melanoma.

REFERENCES

1. Cann SA, van Netten JP, van Netten C. Dr William Coley and tumour regression: a place in history or in the future. Postrgrad Med J 2003;79:672–80.
2. Goldsby RA, Kindt TJ, Osborne BA. Immunology. 4th edition. New York: W.H. Freedman and Company; 2000.
3. American Cancer Society. Melanoma skin cancer. Available at: http://www. cancer.org/cancer/skincancer-melanoma/detailedguide/melanoma-skin-cancer-key-statistics. Accessed August 7, 2014.
4. Smyth MJ. Lloyd John Old 1933-2011. Nature Immunology 2012;13:103.
5. Brandau S, Suttmann H. Thirty years of BCG immunotherapy for non-muscle invasive bladder cancer: a success story with room for improvement. Biomed Pharmacother 2007;61:299–305.
6. Morton DL, Eilber FR, Holmes EC, et al. BCG immunotherapy of malignant melanoma: summary of a seven-year experience. Ann Surg 1974;180(4):635–43.
7. Morton DL, Hsueh EC, Essner R, et al. Prolonged survival of patients receiving active immunotherapy with Canvaxin therapeutic polyvalent vaccine after complete resection of melanoma metastatic to regional lymph nodes. Ann Surg 2002;236(4):438–48 [discussion: 448–9].
8. Kidner TB, Morton DL, Lee DJ, et al. Combined intralesional Bacille Calmette-Guérin (BCG) and topical imiquimod for in-transit melanoma. J Immunother 2012;35(9):716–20.
9. Amin A, White RL. High-dose interleukin-2: is it still indicated for melanoma and RCC in an era of targeted therapies? Oncology 2013;27:680–91.
10. Atkins MB, Lotze MT, Dutcher JP, et al. High-dose recombinant interleukin 2 therapy for patients with metastatic melanoma: analysis of 270 patients treated between 1982 and 1993. J Clin Oncol 1999;17:2105–16.
11. Batus M, Waheed S, Ruby C, et al. Optimal management of metastatic melanoma: current strategies and future directions. Am J Clin Dermatol 2013;14: 179–94.
12. Leach DR, Krummel MF, Allison JP. Enhancement of antitumor immunity by CTLA-4 blockade. Science 1996;271(5256):1734–6.
13. Peggs KS, Quezada SA, Chambers CA, et al. Blockade of CTLA-4 on both effector and regulatory T cell compartments contributes to the antitumor activity of anti-CTLA-4 antibodies. J Exp Med 2009;206(8):1717–25.
14. Simpson TR, Li F, Montalvo-Ortiz W, et al. Fc-dependent depletion of tumor-infiltrating regulatory T cells co-defines the efficacy of anti-CTLA-4 therapy against melanoma. J Exp Med 2013;210(9):1695–710.

15. Hodi FS, O'Day SJ, McDermott DF, et al. Improved survival with ipilimumab in patients with metastatic melanoma. N Engl J Med 2010;363:711–23.
16. Schadendorf D, Hodi FS, Robert C, et al. Pooled analysis of long-term survival data from phase II and phase III trials of ipilimumab in metastatic or locally advanced, unresectable melanoma. Presented at the 2013 European Cancer Congress. Amsterdam, September 27–October 1, 2013.
17. Prieto PA, Yang JC, Sherry RM, et al. CTLA-4 blockade with ipilimumab: long-term follow-up of 177 patients with metastatic melanoma. Clin Cancer Res 2012;18(7): 2039–47.
18. Robert C, Thomas L, Bondarenko I, et al. Ipilimumab plus dacarbazine for previously untreated metastatic melanoma. N Engl J Med 2011;364:2517–26.
19. Wolchok JD, Hoos A, O'Day S, et al. Guidelines for the evaluation of immune therapy activity in solid tumors: immune-related response criteria. Clin Cancer Res 2009;15(23):7412–20.
20. Topalian SL, Hodi FS, Brahmer JR, et al. Safety, activity and immune correlates of anti-PD-1 antibody in cancer. N Engl J Med 2012;366(26):2443–54.
21. Brahmer JR, Tykodi SS, Chow LQ, et al. Safety and activity of anti-PD-L1 antibody in patients with advanced cancer. N Engl J Med 2012;366(26):2455–65.
22. Wolchok JD, Kluger H, Callahan MK, et al. Nivolumab plus ipilimumab in advanced melanoma. N Engl J Med 2013;369(2):122–33.
23. Sznol M, Kluger HM, Callahan MK, et al. Survival, response duration, and activity by BRAF mutation status of nivolumab (NIVO, anti-PD-1, BMS-936558, ONO-4538) and ipilimumab concurrent therapy in advanced melanoma. J Clin Oncol 2014;32(5S Suppl). Abstract: LBA9003.
24. Phan GQ, Rosenberg SA. Adoptive cell transfer for patients with metastatic melanoma: the potential and promise of cancer immunotherapy. Cancer Control 2013;20(4):289–97.
25. Besser MJ, Shapira-Frommer R, Treves AJ, et al. Clinical responses in a phase II study using adoptive transfer of short-term cultured tumor infiltration lymphocytes in metastatic melanoma patients. Clin Cancer Res 2010;16:2646–55.
26. Restifo NP, Dudley ME, Rosenberg SA. Adoptive immunotherapy for cancer: harnessing the T cell response. Nat Rev Immunol 2012;12:269–81.
27. Porter DL, Levine BL, Kalos M, et al. Chimeric antigen receptor-modified T cells in chronic lymphoid leukemia. N Engl J Med 2011;365:725–33.
28. Johnson LA, Morgan RA, Dudley ME, et al. Gene therapy with human and mouse T cell receptors mediates cancer regression and targets normal tissues expressing cognate antigen. Blood 2009;114(3):535–46.
29. Pardoll DM. The blockade of immune checkpoints in cancer immunotherapy. Nat Rev Cancer 2012;12(4):252–64.
30. Vinay DS, Kwon BS. Immunotherapy of cancer with 4-1BB. Mol Cancer Ther 2012;11(5):1062–70.
31. Hirschhorn-Cymerman D, Rizzuto GA, Merghoub T, et al. OX40 engagement and chemotherapy combination provides potent antitumor immunity with concomitant regulatory T cell apoptosis. J Exp Med 2009;206(5):1103–16.
32. Cohen AD, Schaer DA, Liu C, et al. Agonist anti-GITR monoclonal antibody induces melanoma tumor immunity in mice by altering regulatory T cell stability and intra-tumor accumulation. PLoS One 2010;5(5):e10436.
33. Ascierto PA, Simeone E, Sznol M, et al. Clinical experiences with anti-CD137 and anti-PD1 therapeutic antibodies. Semin Oncol 2010;37(5):508–16.
34. Suntharalingam G, Perry MR, Ward S, et al. Cytokine storm in a phase 1 trial of the anti-CD28 monoclonal antibody TGN1412. N Engl J Med 2006;355(10):1018–28.

Targeted Therapies in Melanoma

Stergios J. Moschos, MD[a],*, Ramya Pinnamaneni, MD[b]

KEYWORDS

- Melanoma • Next generation sequencing • BRAF inhibitors • Ocular melanoma
- Immunotherapies

KEY POINTS

- Although melanoma bears one of the highest number of mutations per given DNA length among other malignancies, the most abundant mutations primarily affect 2 major signaling pathways.
- Next-generation sequencing methodologies targeting a panel of cancer-related genes may better capture heterogeneity of melanoma and assist in treatment decisions.
- Several genetic aberrations (mutations, copy number aberrations) can coexist within a particular melanoma, which may be of prognostic and therapeutic significance.
- Although BRAF-mutant melanomas have been the most successful melanoma subset for targeted therapies, progress is ongoing for other melanoma subtypes as well (e.g., RAS mutant, ocular).
- Treatment strategies are more successful in preventing than treating secondary drug resistance; combination treatments among targeted therapies and/or with immunotherapies may be more successful than single-agent approaches.

INTRODUCTION

Similar to those for other cancers, targeted therapies for malignant melanoma (MM) have only been under investigation for a little more than a decade. Before 2010, treatment of MM had achieved minimal progress since the 1970s, when dacarbazine was approved, and when a "one-size-fits-all" approach with various chemotherapeutic approaches had been applied to nearly all cancers. In clinical trial after clinical trial,

This article is funded by NIH (P30-CA016086; NIHMS-ID: 651211).
S.J. Moschos has served as consultant for Genentech, Amgen, and Merck. Dr R. Pinnamaneni has no conflict of interest.
[a] Division of Hematology/Oncology, Department of Medicine, University of North Carolina at Chapel Hill, Physicians Office Building, Suite 3116-CB#7305, 170 Manning Drive, Chapel Hill, NC 27599, USA; [b] Division of Hematology/Oncology, Department of Medicine, East Carolina University, 600 Moye Boulevard, Brody 3E127, Greenville, NC 27834, USA
* Corresponding author.
E-mail address: moschos@med.unc.edu

chemotherapies in MM were proved to be largely ineffective compared with dacarba-zine.[1] In fact, the minimal clinical benefit from systemic treatments was so predictable that clinical efficacy benchmarks were built around the statistical design for future phase II clinical trials in MM.[2] During this frustrating era, few immunotherapies were proved to be promising with durable clinical benefit in a small subset of patients with MM or high risk for relapse melanoma.[1] More than any other time from the past, treatment of MM is currently being shaped around targeted therapies adminis-tered in particular melanoma subgroups, given in precisely defined schedules, alone or in combination with other targeted therapies or various other immunotherapeutic approaches.

A Better Understanding of the Biology of Melanoma Was the Driving Force Behind the Clinical Development of Targeted Therapies

It is becoming increasingly understood that cancers have distinct aberrations in partic-ular cellular processes, in particular DNA repair pathways, which make them either relatively sensitive[3] or refractory[4] to systemic chemotherapies. Melanoma has one of the highest mutation frequencies[5] and frequently shows elevated expression of DNA repair proteins.[6] Four important points are remarkable with respect to genetic aberrations in melanoma:

1. Only a handful of genes are more frequently mutated (**Fig. 1**) or show gene copy number alterations (amplifications or deletions, **Fig. 2**) than others,[7,8] whereas the clinical importance of most other genetic aberrations is currently unclear.
2. Although most frequently mutated genes bear mutational "hotspots" ("canonical" mutations), increasing evidence suggests the presence of noncanonical mutations (see **Fig. 1**) that can only be identified using next-generation sequencing methodologies.
3. The most frequently mutated genes are components of 2 principal signaling path-ways, the Ras–Raf–MEK–ERK and the PI3K–mTOR signaling pathway (**Fig. 3**). The activation status of these kinases within each of these pathways is not independent from each other and dynamically adjusts to environmental changes, including tar-geted treatments.[9]
4. The most frequently occurring mutations BRAF and RAS proteins are paradoxically not related to sun exposure, can be found in early stages of melanoma, or even pre-malignant conditions,[10] and are retained during later stages of melanoma.[11]
5. More than 1 mutation and/or gene copy alteration can coexist within a melanoma, which can have important clinical implications (see **Figs. 1** and **2**).[12]
6. Response to immunotherapies is independent from mutational status.[13]

In preliminary analyses of mutations of more than 350 cutaneous melanoma spec-imens as part of the Cancer Genome Atlas, cutaneous melanomas can be convention-ally classified in 4 different mutational groups (see **Fig. 1**)[8]:

1. "Hotspot" mutations in the BRAFV600 as well as immediately adjacent codons;
2. "Hotspot" mutations of the RAS oncogenes (N-, K-, or H-RAS) with the predomi-nance of those occurring in NRAS (>90%);
3. Mutations of the neurofibromatosis 1 gene (NF1), an inhibitor of RAS signaling (**Fig. 4**) without any concurrent hotspot mutations in the BRAF and NRAS (approx-imately 10%); and
4. No mutations in any of these genes.

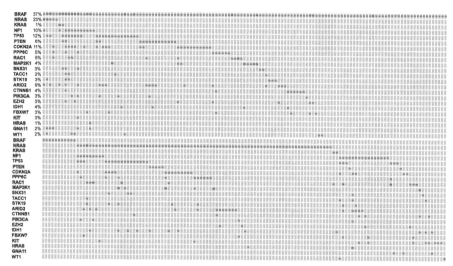

Fig. 1. Frequency of somatic mutations that were previously identified in the work presented in the Hodis and colleagues[7] article and applied in the publicly available cohort of cutaneous melanoma samples that has been collected as part of the Cancer Genome Atlas Project. Only 257 out of the so far (August 17, 2014) analyzed 375 samples that bear mutations (*green dots*) in any of these genes are shown. Neurofibromatosis 1 gene (NF1), HRAS, and KRAS are also presented to emphasize the 4 emerging subgroups on the basis of BRAF, RAS, and NF1 mutations, versus no mutation (triple wild-type group). Mutations highlighted with red border signify noncanonical mutations. Most genes, highlighted in red, are components of the BRAF/MEK/ERK, or PI3K/Akt signaling (see **Fig. 3** for further details). Analysis was performed using the cBioportal for Cancer Genomics (www.cbioportal.org) in compliance with early publication of results from the website, as per Cerami and colleagues[59] and Gao and colleagues.[60]

TREATING PATIENTS WITH MALIGNANT MELANOMA IN THE ERA OF SMALL MOLECULE INHIBITORS

The approach to a patient with MM has dramatically changed since 2010 with the advent of small inhibitor therapies, especially for BRAF-mutant patients. In addition to factors such as patient performance status, tumor doubling time, ability to perform

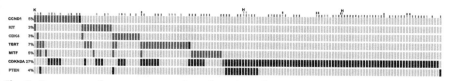

Fig. 2. Frequency of gene copy number alterations that were previously identified in the work presented in the Hodis and colleagues[7] and applied in the publicly available cohort of cutaneous melanoma samples that has been collected as part of the Cancer Genome Atlas Project. Only 145 out of the so far (August 17, 2014) analyzed 375 sample that bear gene amplifications (*red bars*), or gene deletions (*blue bars*) in any of these genes are shown. Samples with BRAF (*red dots*), RAS (*green dots*), or neurofibromatosis 1 gene (NF1; *purple dots*) mutations are also shown for associations. Analysis was performed using the cBioportal for Cancer Genomics (www.cbioportal.org) in compliance with early publication of results from the website, as per Cerami and colleagues[59] and Gao and colleagues.[60]

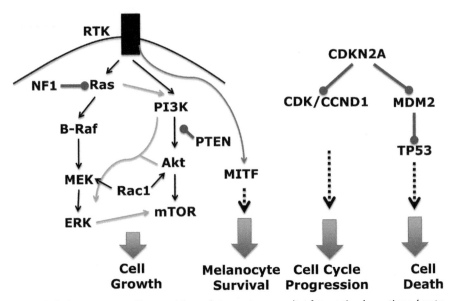

Fig. 3. Cellular processes disrupted in melanoma as a result of genetic aberrations (mutations or gene copy number alterations). See **Figs. 1** and **2** for details regarding the type and frequency of genetic aberrations. Red lines indicate inhibition; blue and black indicate activation. mTOR, mammalian target of rapamycin; PTEN, protein tyrosine phosphatase; RTK, receptor tyrosine kinase.

metastatectomy, comorbid factors, American Joint Committee on Cancer (AJCC) staging system guidelines, knowledge about the mutation status for at least BRAF, NRAS, and KIT is becoming the standard of care for prognostic[14] and treatment reasons. Next-generation sequencing methodologies with the ability to sequence several hundred cancer-associated genes are increasingly being incorporated into standard

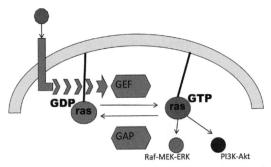

Fig. 4. Simplified diagram on the regulation of the RAS superfamily of small GTPases and the role of neurofibromatosis 1 gene (NF1). RAS proteins become active versus inactive if bound to GTP and GDP, respectively. Extracellular growth factor signals (*red circle*) are transmitted through growth factor receptors (*light blue*) to guanine nucleotide exchange factors (GEF), which activate RAS (*red*) by exchanging GDP for GTP. In contrast, GTPase activating proteins, including NF1, tend to keep RAS proteins in their inactive state (*light blue*). Please note the promiscuity of RAS signaling, which activate several signaling pathways, including the MAPK as well as the PI3K-Akt pathway.

therapeutic decisions and so far have revealed that the mutational landscape of melanoma is more complex than was originally thought.[15]

Metastatectomy remains the best treatment for patients who can become completely free of distant metastatic disease with surgery.[16] However, controversies exist with respect to the optimal sequencing of systemic therapies for patients with unresectable MM. Retrospective analysis of BRAF-mutant patients who participated in the European Ipilimumab Expanded Access program suggest that the overall survival of patients with BRAF-mutant melanoma who originally received a single-agent mitogen-activated protein kinase (MAPK) inhibitor (MAPKi) followed by ipilimumab was inferior to that of patients who received ipilimumab first, followed by MAPKi.[13] Current guidelines suggest that in the absence of a clinical trial, patients with relatively asymptomatic, slow tumor kinetics, M1a/M1b disease—all presumed surrogate factors of a relatively more functional host immune system—should be initially considered for an immunotherapy followed by targeted therapy, if available, or chemotherapy.

TREATMENT WITH SINGLE-AGENT TARGETED AGENTS
All 3 US Food and Drug Administration–Approved Targeted Therapies in Metastatic Melanoma are for Patients with BRAF-Mutant Melanoma

As of May 2013 there are 3 US Food and Drug Administration (FDA)-approved MAPKi for MM: the 2 BRAF inhibitors (BRAFi), vemurafenib and dabrafenib, and the first-in-class MEK inhibitor (MEKi), trametinib. Their approval was based on randomized, phase III trials in which each of the investigational agents was compared against dacarbazine for patients with unresectable BRAFV600E(K)-mutant MM.[17–19] All important clinical endpoints were in favor of the investigational agents. Five key observations were remarkable:

1. Responses were seen early during treatment, suggesting direct antitumor effect. However, further investigation showed that BRAFi may actually have effects on the tumor microenvironment, such as increased influx of effector CD8[+] cells infiltrating the tumor,[20] upregulation of immune checkpoint proteins within the tumor,[21] and suppression of angiogenic molecules, such as vascular endothelial growth factor.[22] These effects may be either secondary to suppression of downstream actions of BRAF oncogenic signaling within melanoma cells themselves, or secondary to paradoxical activation of BRAF signaling within immune cells.[23]
2. Although antitumor responses have been impressive, the majority of responses were partial. Early studies using novel proteomic methods from analysis of the adaptive responses of the kinome in various melanoma cell lines following treatment with single-agent BRAFi or MEKi[24] reveal incomplete suppression of the activity of all components of the RAF–MEK1/2–ERK pathway.[25]
3. Development of secondary resistance was seen in the majority of patients. Although general mechanisms of resistance are described elsewhere in this article, a surrogate clinical marker for durable responses to BRAFi was the ability to achieve complete antitumor response.[26,27]
4. All 3 treatments are administered orally and overall well tolerated with side effects similar to other, previously FDA-approved tyrosine kinase inhibitors. The most interesting class-specific side effect was the small but significantly higher incidence of cutaneous squamous carcinomas, especially when preexisting skin lesions bear KRAS or HRAS mutations.[28] Side effects from trametinib include high blood pressure, diarrhea, bleeding, coagulopathies, cardiomyopathy, and ocular toxicities.

5. All trials were conducted in patients with extracranial MM. Nevertheless, phase II trials using BRAFi in patients with active brain metastases showed considerable intracranial antitumor responses.[29,30] These results were somewhat unexpected in view of the fact that none of the 3 agents achieves significant drug levels within the central nervous system in preclinical studies (Vaidhyanathan and collegues,[31] and references therein). The mechanism for such an antitumor effect within the brain is, currently unknown, but it is reasonable to speculate that the blood–brain barrier is to a certain extent, compromised allowing for drug to enter the brain, a hypothesis that is currently being clinically tested (ClinicalTrials.gov Identifier NCT01978236).

Non–US Food and Drug Administration-Approved but Promising Therapies for Patients with Malignant Melanoma: More Mitogen-Activated Protein Kinase Pathway Inhibitors, Other Pathways, and Effects on Other Melanoma Subtypes

Do other BRAF inhibitors have a role in BRAF-mutant melanoma?
Encorafenib (LGX818) is the third BRAFi in advanced stages of clinical development. In contrast with other BRAFi, encorafenib has an extremely long dissociation half-life (30 hours vs 2 and 0.5 hours for dabrafenib and vemurafenib, respectively), a property that makes encorafenib extremely potent. In line with these preclinical data, a phase I trial of single-agent encorafenib in patients with BRAF-mutant MM showed that antitumor responses were also seen among patients who have previously received BRAFi,[32] suggesting that prolonged inhibition of the target may further improve therapeutic benefit.

Treatment of patients with NRAS-mutant melanoma
NRAS-mutant melanomas have an overall worse prognosis than the more abundant BRAF-mutant melanomas.[14] This is attributed to the relative "promiscuity" of the RAS family of proteins to signal through multiple signaling pathways, including the MAPK and the PI3K/Akt pathway, as opposed to RAF proteins that are relatively more committed to signal through the MAPK pathway (see **Fig. 3**).[33] Owing to difficulties in developing direct RAS inhibitors, current efforts focus on inhibiting druggable downstream effectors of RAS proteins, such as MEK. A phase II trial of binimetinib (MEK162), a highly specific MEKi, in patients with NRAS-mutant melanoma showed an approximately 20% partial response,[34] a promising result that is currently being investigated in a large, randomized, phase III trial (NCT01763164). Of note, no responses were seen with trametinib.[35]

Targeting mutations in rare melanomas
cKIT is a type III transmembrane receptor tyrosine kinase that mediates signaling via various pathways and plays an important physiologic role in the development and maintenance of various cells, including melanocytes. A number of genetic aberrations of the cKIT gene have been observed in melanoma from both cutaneous (acral and chronically sun damaged skin) and mucosal primary, including mutations in particular exons (eg, 11 and 13) and gene amplifications.[36] Recently reported trials using various cKIT inhibitors focusing on melanomas that bear cKIT genetic aberrations are proof-of-principle that melanomas driven by constitutively active proto-oncogenes can be successfully targeted by small molecule inhibitor therapies. These trials show that antitumor responses can occur, particularly in patients with activating mutations, as opposed to gene amplifications, and can occasionally be durable.[36]

Over the last few years, significant advances have been made toward understanding the biology of ocular melanoma. Primary ocular melanomas frequently bear activating, mutually exclusive hotspot mutations in 2 of the guanine nucleotide-binding proteins for Aq and A11 (GNAQ and GNA11),[37] which lead to constitutive activation of phospholipase C β and MAPK. In addition, approximately one-half of primary uveal melanomas bear inactivating mutations in the BRCA1-associated protein 1 (BAP1), a genetic event that usually follows that of GNAQ/GNA11, and is associated with propensity for distant metastases.[38] Early clinical trials suggest that targeting ocular melanomas with MEKi is associated with better clinical benefit compared with standard chemotherapy,[39] a result that is currently being confirmed in a large, phase III trial (NCT01974752). A phase I clinical trial of a novel phospholipase C β inhibitor, AEB071, in patients with ocular melanoma showed early promising safety and efficacy results.[40] The role of other targeted treatments against ocular melanoma with BAP1 mutation is currently under investigation (NCT01587352).

THERAPIES USING COMBINATIONS OF SMALL MOLECULE INHIBITORS
Combinations Among Small Molecule Inhibitors

Concurrent suppression of BRAF plus MEK results in more potent and sustained suppression of ERK signaling, presumably owing to incomplete suppression of the MAPK pathway by either agent alone.[25] In fact, treatment of patients with BRAFV600E,K-mutant MM with dabrafenib and trametinib (D+T) led to a higher incidence of complete antitumor responses.[41] In line with this, the combination of D+T was associated with more prolonged, progression-free survival compared with dabrafenib alone in a randomized, phase III trial, COMBI-d.[42] In this trial, D+T was well tolerated overall, with lesser frequency of keratoacanthomas and squamous cell carcinomas, although significant pyrexia, more frequent dose reductions, interruptions, and permanent discontinuations were observed in the D+T compared with dabrafenib alone arm. Nevertheless, the safety and efficacy data led to the FDA approval of D+T as a frontline therapy for patients with BRAFV600E,K-mutant melanoma. Randomized, phase III trials testing the efficacy of concurrent BRAF plus MEK inhibition with other BRAFi+MEKi are underway.[43,44]

Given the high incidence of NRAS mutations that coexist with CDKN2A locus genetic aberrations[7,8] and the strong preclinical rationale to combine MEK plus CDK inhibitors in NRAS-driven genetically engineered mouse models,[45] a clinical trial of combined MEKi and CDK inhibition using binimetinib plus LEE011 is underway. Preliminary results suggest that this treatment combination induces antitumor responses in approximately one-third of the analyzed patients, although dosing schedules in relation to toxicity and tolerability are currently being addressed.[46]

Combinations of Small Molecule Inhibitors and Immunotherapies

It is becoming increasingly understood that small molecule inhibitor therapies and immunotherapies have complementary strengths and limitations[47] and various preclinical models have suggested a synergistic mechanism of action between these 2 treatment modalities.[23,48,49] Current treatment combinations are being tested in BRAF-mutant patients, given the lack of effective targeted therapies in other groups. Scheduling of these treatments—concurrent versus sequential—as well as selection of optimal drug combinations is important not only to minimize toxicity, but also to avoid potential small molecule inhibitor-mediated immunosuppression,[50] and to optimize the treatment effect granted by each drug. Despite early concerns that this combination could be associated with considerable toxicity, early results from subsequent ongoing trials suggest that the observed toxicities may not be only drug class effect, but also related to the particular drug combination tested.[51] As these and other trials (NCT01656642 and NCT01988896) mature, and even evolve into large, randomized studies in the near future, we will be able to better assess durability of responses, a clinical benefit that is infrequently shared among targeted therapies.

TREATMENT RESISTANCE

Based on the history of targeted therapies in other malignancies, resistance to targeted therapies in melanoma was highly expected. Several excellent reviews have been written for this important topic.[52] In the case of BRAF-mutant melanoma, the most extensively studied subtype with respect to drug resistance, these mechanisms may or may not involve reactivation of the ERK signaling pathway. In fact, on most occasions BRAF-mutant, MAPKi-resistant melanoma remain "addicted" to MAPK signaling, which explains why the overall survival of patients who continue to be treated beyond disease progression with MAPKi is significantly longer compared with those who switch to non–MAPKi-based treatments.[53] Another important aspect is the role of PI3K/Akt signaling in primary as well as secondary drug resistance, either via acquired genetic alteration or secondary activation of the pathway by endogenous (RAS) or environmental factors.[54,55] So far, approaches to overcome resistance after it is developed have been challenging, and current efforts focus on prevention of drug resistance. It is anticipated that small molecule inhibitors with superior pharmacodynamic properties (eg, encorafenib) and/or addition of a third targeted therapy to the BRAF/MEKi backbone may overcome the challenge of turning the drugs' cell inhibitory effect to an actual cell killing one. While trials testing combinations of 3 small molecule inhibitors are underway (eg, NCT02110355), toxicity and tolerability will be a significant concern, in addition to efficacy. This is a particular concern when MAPKi were previously combined with inhibitors of the PI3K/Akt pathway.[56]

DISCUSSION

Although great progress has been achieved toward finding effective treatments for patients with BRAF-mutant melanoma, therapeutic advances are only beginning to occur in RAS-mutant melanoma. The biology of melanomas that bear no oncogenic mutations for BRAF/RAS has only recently begun to be systematically investigated,[57] but the subgroup that bears NF1 mutations, which is negative inhibitor of RAS signaling,[58] suggests that an even greater proportion of melanomas than what was originally thought may actually be addicted to RAS or RAF/MEK signaling. Clearly, targeted therapies provide a clinical benefit that is only durable in a small subset of patients. Nevertheless, the remarkable ability of small molecule inhibitors to suppress tumor growth leads to a better functioning immune system dysfunction, which, even if only temporary, may pave the way for better and more durable responses using immunotherapies. The tremendous efficacy of such targeted therapies in distant MM is already being investigated in earlier stages of disease, where the risk of relapse is high (NCT1682083 and 01667419). It is actually the administration of such treatments at an earlier stage that is expected to significantly change the natural history of disease over the next decade, especially the development of challenging future complications that are inherently difficult to treat (eg, brain metastases).

Finally, the notion of "targeted" therapies may likely be further expanded in the near future, thanks to projects such as the Cancer Genome Atlas. As part of this project, clinicopathologically well-annotated, snap-frozen tumors undergo profiling across multiple molecular data platforms for downstream integrative bioinformatics analysis (DNA and RNA sequencing as well as microRNA, methylation, and proteomic profiling). This high-order investigation will most likely identify important nongenetic "targets" amenable to therapeutic manipulation.[8]

REFERENCES

1. Lee C, Collichio F, Ollila D, et al. Historical review of melanoma treatment and outcomes. Clin Dermatol 2013;31:141–7.
2. Korn EL, Liu PY, Lee SJ, et al. Meta-analysis of phase II cooperative group trials in metastatic stage IV melanoma to determine progression-free and overall survival benchmarks for future phase II trials. J Clin Oncol 2008;26:527–34.
3. Cancer Genome Atlas Network. Comprehensive molecular portraits of human breast tumours. Nature 2012;490:61–70.
4. Cancer Genome Atlas Research Network. Comprehensive molecular characterization of clear cell renal cell carcinoma. Nature 2013;499:43–9.
5. Alexandrov LB, Nik-Zainal S, Wedge DC, et al. Signatures of mutational processes in human cancer. Nature 2013;500:415–21.
6. Jewell R, Conway C, Mitra A, et al. Patterns of expression of DNA repair genes and relapse from melanoma. Clin Cancer Res 2010;16:5211–21.
7. Hodis E, Watson IR, Kryukov GV, et al. A landscape of driver mutations in melanoma. Cell 2012;150:251–63.
8. Watson I. Comprehensive molecular characterization of regional metastatic melanoma. Oral presentation at The Cancer Genome Atlas 3rd Annual Scientific Symposium, May 12-13. National Institutes of Health, Bethesda, MD, 2014.
9. Johnson GL, Stuhlmiller TJ, Angus SP, et al. Molecular pathways: adaptive kinome reprogramming in response to targeted inhibition of the BRAF-MEK-ERK pathway in cancer. Clin Cancer Res 2014;20:2516–22.
10. Poynter JN, Elder JT, Fullen DR, et al. BRAF and NRAS mutations in melanoma and melanocytic nevi. Melanoma Res 2006;16:267–73.
11. Colombino M, Capone M, Lissia A, et al. BRAF/NRAS mutation frequencies among primary tumors and metastases in patients with melanoma. J Clin Oncol 2012;30:2522–9.
12. Nathanson KL, Martin AM, Wubbenhorst B, et al. Tumor genetic analyses of patients with metastatic melanoma treated with the BRAF inhibitor dabrafenib (GSK2118436). Clin Cancer Res 2013;19:4868–78.
13. Ascierto PA, Simeone E, Sileni VC, et al. Clinical experience with ipilimumab 3 mg/kg: real-world efficacy and safety data from an expanded access programme cohort. J Transl Med 2014;12:116.
14. Jakob JA, Bassett RL Jr, Ng CS, et al. NRAS mutation status is an independent prognostic factor in metastatic melanoma. Cancer 2012;118:4014–23.
15. Jeck WR, Parker J, Carson CC, et al. Targeted next generation sequencing identifies clinically actionable mutations in patients with melanoma. Pigment Cell Melanoma Res 2014;27:653–63.
16. Sosman JA, Moon J, Tuthill RJ, et al. A phase 2 trial of complete resection for stage IV melanoma: results of Southwest Oncology Group Clinical Trial S9430. Cancer 2011;117:4740–6.
17. McArthur GA, Chapman PB, Robert C, et al. Safety and efficacy of vemurafenib in BRAF(V600E) and BRAF(V600K) mutation-positive melanoma (BRIM-3): extended follow-up of a phase 3, randomised, open-label study. Lancet Oncol 2014;15:323–32.
18. Hauschild A, Grob JJ, Demidov LV, et al. Dabrafenib in BRAF-mutated metastatic melanoma: a multicentre, open-label, phase 3 randomised controlled trial. Lancet 2012;380:358–65.
19. Flaherty KT, Robert C, Hersey P, et al. Improved survival with MEK inhibition in BRAF-mutated melanoma. N Engl J Med 2012;367:107–14.

20. Wilmott JS, Long GV, Howle JR, et al. Selective BRAF inhibitors induce marked T-cell infiltration into human metastatic melanoma. Clin Cancer Res 2012;18: 1386–94.
21. Frederick DT, Piris A, Cogdill AP, et al. BRAF inhibition is associated with enhanced melanoma antigen expression and a more favorable tumor microenvironment in patients with metastatic melanoma. Clin Cancer Res 2013;19: 1225–31.
22. Khalili JS, Liu S, Rodriguez-Cruz TG, et al. Oncogenic BRAF(V600E) promotes stromal cell-mediated immunosuppression via induction of interleukin-1 in melanoma. Clin Cancer Res 2012;18:5329–40.
23. Koya RC, Mok S, Otte N, et al. BRAF inhibitor vemurafenib improves the antitumor activity of adoptive cell immunotherapy. Cancer Res 2012;72:3928–37.
24. Duncan JS, Whittle MC, Nakamura K, et al. Dynamic reprogramming of the kinome in response to targeted MEK inhibition in triple-negative breast cancer. Cell 2012;149:307–21.
25. Angus SP, Stuhlmiller TJ, Reuther R, et al. Defining the adaptive kinome response to BRAF and MEK inhibition in melanoma (abstr 4761). AACR Annual Meeting, April 5-9. San Diego, CA, 2014.
26. Kim K, Amaravadi RK, Flaherty KT, et al. Significant long-term survival benefit demonstrated with vemurafenib in ongoing phase I study. Presented in the Society of Melanoma Research Annual Meeting, Nov 8-11. Hollywood, CA, 2012.
27. Flaherty KT, Puzanov I, Kim KB, et al. Inhibition of mutated, activated BRAF in metastatic melanoma. N Engl J Med 2010;363:809–19.
28. Su F, Viros A, Milagre C, et al. RAS mutations in cutaneous squamous-cell carcinomas in patients treated with BRAF inhibitors. N Engl J Med 2012;366:207–15.
29. Long GV, Trefzer U, Davies MA, et al. Dabrafenib in patients with Val600Glu or Val600Lys BRAF-mutant melanoma metastatic to the brain (BREAK-MB): a multicentre, open-label, phase 2 trial. Lancet Oncol 2012;13:1087–95.
30. Dummer R, Goldinger SM, Turtschi CP, et al. Vemurafenib in patients with BRAF(V600) mutation-positive melanoma with symptomatic brain metastases: final results of an open-label pilot study. Eur J Cancer 2014;50:611–21.
31. Vaidhyanathan S, Mittapalli RK, Sarkaria JN, et al. Factors influencing the CNS distribution of a novel MEK-1/2 inhibitor: implications for combination therapy for melanoma brain metastases. Drug Metab Dispos 2014;42:1292–300.
32. Dummer R, Robert C, Nyakas M, et al. Initial results from a phase I, open-label, dose escalation study of the oral BRAF inhibitor LGX818 in patients with BRAF V600 mutant advanced or metastatic melanoma (abstr 9028). ASCO Annual Meeting, May 31-June 2. Chicago, IL, 2013.
33. Rodriguez-Viciana P, Sabatier C, McCormick F. Signaling specificity by Ras family GTPases is determined by the full spectrum of effectors they regulate. Mol Cell Biol 2004;24:4943–54.
34. Ascierto PA, Schadendorf D, Berking C, et al. MEK162 for patients with advanced melanoma harbouring NRAS or Val600 BRAF mutations: a non-randomised, open-label phase 2 study. Lancet Oncol 2013;14:249–56.
35. Falchook GS, Lewis KD, Infante JR, et al. Activity of the oral MEK inhibitor trametinib in patients with advanced melanoma: a phase 1 dose-escalation trial. Lancet Oncol 2012;13:782–9.
36. Curtin JA, Busam K, Pinkel D, et al. Somatic activation of KIT in distinct subtypes of melanoma. J Clin Oncol 2006;24:4340–6.
37. Van Raamsdonk CD, Griewank KG, Crosby MB, et al. Mutations in GNA11 in uveal melanoma. N Engl J Med 2010;363:2191–9.

38. Harbour JW, Onken MD, Roberson ED, et al. Frequent mutation of BAP1 in metastasizing uveal melanomas. Science 2010;330:1410–3.
39. Carvajal RD, Sosman JA, Quevedo JF, et al. Effect of selumetinib vs chemotherapy on progression-free survival in uveal melanoma: a randomized clinical trial. JAMA 2014;311:2397–405.
40. Piperno-Neumann S, Kapiteijn E, Larkin JM, et al. Phase I dose-escalation study of the protein kinase C inhibitor AEB071 in patients with metastatic uveal melanoma (abstr 9030). ASCO Annual Meeting. Chicago, IL, 2014.
41. Flaherty KT, Infante JR, Daud A, et al. Combined BRAF and MEK inhibition in melanoma with BRAF V600 mutations. N Engl J Med 2012;367:1694–703.
42. Long GV, Stroyakovskiy D, Gogas H, et al. Combined BRAF and MEK inhibition versus BRAF inhibition alone in melanoma. N Engl J Med 2014;371:1877–88.
43. Ribas A, Gonzalez R, Pavlick A, et al. Combination of vemurafenib and cobimetinib in patients with advanced BRAF(V600)-mutated melanoma: a phase 1b study. Lancet Oncol 2014;15:954–65.
44. Kefford R, Miller WH, Tan DS, et al. Preliminary results from a phase Ib/II, open-label, dose-escalation study of the oral BRAF inhibitor LGX818 in combination with the oral MEK1/2 inhibitor MEK162 in BRAF V600-dependent advanced solid tumors (abstr 9029). ASCO Annual Meeting, May 31-June 2. Chicago, IL, 2013.
45. Kwong LN, Costello JC, Liu H, et al. Oncogenic NRAS signaling differentially regulates survival and proliferation in melanoma. Nat Med 2012;18:1503–10.
46. Sosman JA, Kittaneh M, Lolkema MP, et al. A phase 1b/2 study of LEE011 in combination with binimetinib (MEK162) in patients with NRAS-mutant melanoma: Early encouraging clinical activity (abstr 9009). In ASCO (ed): ASCO 2014 Annual Meeting, May 30-June 3. Chicago, IL.
47. Ribas A, Hersey P, Middleton MR, et al. New challenges in endpoints for drug development in advanced melanoma. Clin Cancer Res 2012;18:336–41.
48. Mok S, Koya RC, Tsui C, et al. Inhibition of CSF-1 receptor improves the antitumor efficacy of adoptive cell transfer immunotherapy. Cancer Res 2014;74:153–61.
49. Liu C, Peng W, Xu C, et al. BRAF inhibition increases tumor infiltration by T cells and enhances the antitumor activity of adoptive immunotherapy in mice. Clin Cancer Res 2013;19:393–403.
50. Boni A, Cogdill AP, Dang P, et al. Selective BRAFV600E inhibition enhances T-cell recognition of melanoma without affecting lymphocyte function. Cancer Res 2010;70:5213–9.
51. Puzanov I, Callahan MK, Linette GP, et al. Phase 1 study of the BRAF inhibitor dabrafenib with or without the MEK inhibitor trametinib in combination with ipilimumab for V600E/K mutation–positive unresectable or metastatic melanoma (abstr 2511), ASCO Annual Meeting, May 30-June 3. Chicago, IL, 2014.
52. Lito P, Rosen N, Solit DB. Tumor adaptation and resistance to RAF inhibitors. Nat Med 2013;19:1401–9.
53. Chan MM, Haydu LE, Menzies AM, et al. The nature and management of metastatic melanoma after progression on BRAF inhibitors: effects of extended BRAF inhibition. Cancer 2014;120:3142–53.
54. Shi H, Hong A, Kong X, et al. A novel AKT1 mutant amplifies an adaptive melanoma response to BRAF inhibition. Cancer Discov 2014;4:69–79.
55. Trunzer K, Pavlick AC, Schuchter L, et al. Pharmacodynamic effects and mechanisms of resistance to vemurafenib in patients with metastatic melanoma. J Clin Oncol 2013;31:1767–74.

56. Algazi AP, Posch C, Ortiz-Urda S, et al. A phase I trial of BKM120 combined with vemurafenib in BRAFV600E/k mutant advanced melanoma (abstr 9101), ASCO Annual Meeting, May 30-June 3. Chicago, IL, 2014.

57. Mar VJ, Wong SQ, Li J, et al. BRAF/NRAS wild-type melanomas have a high mutation load correlating with histologic and molecular signatures of UV damage. Clin Cancer Res 2013;19:4589–98.

58. Nissan MH, Pratilas CA, Jones AM, et al. Loss of NF1 in cutaneous melanoma is associated with RAS activation and MEK dependence. Cancer Res 2014;74:2340–50.

59. Cerami E, Gao J, Dogrusoz U, et al. The cBio cancer genomics portal: an open platform for exploring multidimensional cancer genomics data. Cancer Discov 2012;2:401–4.

60. Gao J, Aksoy BA, Dogrusoz U, et al. Integrative analysis of complex cancer genomics and clinical profiles using the cBioPortal. Sci Signal 2013;6:pl1.

Long-term Follow-up for Melanoma Patients

Is There Any Evidence of a Benefit?

Natasha M. Rueth, MD, MS, Kate D. Cromwell, MS, MPH,
Janice N. Cormier, MD, MPH*

KEYWORDS

- Evidence-based surveillance • Cost-effectiveness • Melanoma • Survivorship
- Guidelines • Diagnostic imaging

KEY POINTS

- Current surveillance practices for melanoma are based on low-level evidence with unknown clinical impact.
- Surveillance for melanoma recurrence is most frequently based on preferences of patient and provider.
- Serial routine surveillance imaging has demonstrated limited evidence for detecting recurrent melanoma at a time in which it is treatable.

INTRODUCTION

Contemporary surveillance guidelines for cancer survivors are low-level, category 2A to 2B recommendations (ie, "based upon lower-level evidence, there is *uniform consensus* [category 2A] or *consensus* [category 2B] that the intervention is appropriate")[1] and therefore heavily depend on expert opinion. Even the handful of tumor types for which surveillance recommendations have been rigorously studied lack category 1 (ie, "based upon high-level evidence, there is uniform consensus that the intervention is appropriate")[1] surveillance recommendations. As an example, seven clinical trials[2–8] have evaluated various surveillance regimens for patients with surgically treated colorectal cancer and yielded mixed results. Subsequent meta-analyses of

The Authors have nothing to disclose.
Department of Surgical Oncology, The University of Texas MD Anderson Cancer Center, Unit 1484, 1400 Holcombe Boulevard, Houston, TX 77230-1402, USA
* Corresponding author.
E-mail address: jcormier@mdanderson.org

Surg Oncol Clin N Am 24 (2015) 359–377
http://dx.doi.org/10.1016/j.soc.2014.12.012
1055-3207/15/$ – see front matter © 2015 Elsevier Inc. All rights reserved.

these results[9,10] have suggested improvements in overall survival (but not disease-specific survival) in the setting of intensive surveillance. In contrast, several well-designed randomized studies evaluating surveillance strategies of varying intensities for women with treated breast cancer have shown no survival benefit for intensive surveillance compared with less intensive strategies.[11–14] Still, controversy regarding breast cancer surveillance exists, and surveillance practice patterns vary widely.

From a practical perspective, the frequency and intensity of follow-up for cancer survivors are determined by the resources available and the preferences of the patient in conjunction with a provider's specific preferences. These factors have increasingly important implications as the number of cancer survivors in the world increases. Because of improvements in the detection of early stage melanoma at a time when adequate local treatment is potentially curative, 5-year relative survival rates for patients with melanoma now exceed 90%,[15] which means that more people are living longer after the diagnosis of what was once a frequently deadly cancer.[16] However, in the absence of evidence-based follow-up guidelines, the question is how can clinicians best manage melanoma cases to detect disease recurrence while it is still treatable?

Half of all patients treated for melanoma have a recurrence.[17,18] Of these recurrences, approximately 50% are in the regional lymph nodes, 20% are local recurrences, and 30% arise at distant sites.[19–21] Although most recurrences develop in the first 2 to 3 years after treatment, some late recurrences more than 10 years after treatment are well documented, particularly for patients who initially had early stage melanoma. In a retrospective study of more than 7100 patients with early stage melanoma, Crowley and Seigler[22] reported that the overall rate of recurrence 10 years after the diagnosis of the primary was 2.4%. Surgical resection is generally performed for local and regional recurrences, with good survival outcome, and metastasectomy for distant recurrences in very carefully selected patients has demonstrated survival benefits.[23–26]

In designing optimal surveillance strategies, clinicians must focus on the risk of early recurrence but must also consider the risk of late recurrences within the context of a patient's changing risk over time. As an example, in a retrospective study of 340 patients with stage III melanoma, Romano and colleagues[27] found that most local and regional recurrences were detected by physical examination alone, whereas patients with distant recurrences most frequently presented with symptoms. Routine computed tomography (CT) imaging detected asymptomatic recurrences in 25% of all patients studied, often within 3 years of the original melanoma diagnosis.[27] In this study, the incidence of a first-time distant recurrence was 5% or less after 32 months, 40 months, and 21 months for patients with stage IIIA, IIIB, and IIIC disease, respectively, leading the authors to conclude that routine CT imaging as a surveillance method would have low yield beyond those time points.[27]

Importantly, because cancer survival estimates are heavily influenced by early cancer deaths, the estimates may not accurately reflect long-term outcomes for patients who survive to a certain point after the original diagnosis. As an alternative approach to predicting long-term survival, conditional survival analysis calculates the changing risk of death over time. For patients with all stages of melanoma, conditional survival studies have demonstrated that survival estimates improve dramatically as survival time increases, such that eventually, the original stage at diagnosis is no longer a significant predictor of ongoing survival (**Fig. 1**).[21,22] These two competing concepts—indolent disease with the potential for late recurrences but in light of known improvements in cancer survival as time from original treatment increases—make optimal melanoma surveillance a complex challenge for patients and clinicians.

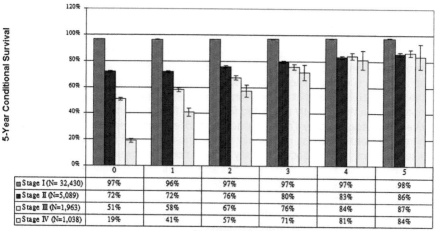

5-Year Conditional Survival	0	1	2	3	4	5
▨ Stage I (N= 32,430)	97%	96%	97%	97%	97%	98%
▪ Stage II (N=5,089)	72%	72%	76%	80%	83%	86%
▢ Stage III (N=1,963)	51%	58%	67%	76%	84%	87%
▢ Stage IV (N=1,038)	19%	41%	57%	71%	81%	84%

Years Alive After Diagnosis

Fig. 1. Melanoma-specific 5-year conditional survival estimates stratified by disease stage. (*From* Xing Y, Chang GJ, Hu CY, et al. Conditional survival estimates improve over time for patients with advanced melanoma: results from a population-based analysis. Cancer 2010;116(9):2237, with permission.)

To address these challenges, current guidelines for surveillance in patients with melanoma published by the National Comprehensive Cancer Network[1] emphasize more frequent visits with more intensive stage-specific surveillance imaging early in the posttreatment phase, when the risk of recurrence is greatest. As the disease-free interval increases, office visits and imaging should become less frequent, but annual skin examinations for all stages of primary disease should continue for the rest of the patient's life. Annual skin examinations for life, particularly for patients with early stage, low-risk melanoma, are a logical surveillance strategy based on recurrence and survival patterns; however, recommendations become less clear for patients with locally advanced stage III melanoma. Beyond annual skin examinations, the current recommendations for patients with stage III melanoma range from conventional x-ray radiography of the chest to a complex positron emission tomography (PET)/CT scan at time intervals ranging from 3 to 12 months.

The data available to aid in the development of appropriate stage-specific surveillance recommendations are limited in scope and value. The broad generalities in surveillance recommendations very likely reflect uncertainties in modern resource use and a limited understanding of the effects of different surveillance strategies on patient quality of life and cancer survival. Toward elucidating these uncertainties and enhancing the understanding of the effects of surveillance strategies on quality of life and survival for patients with melanoma, this article reviews issues key to designing surveillance strategies, including early detection, surveillance evaluation modalities, surveillance effectiveness, variation in current surveillance practices, surveillance costs, and other practice implications.

BENEFITS OF EARLY DETECTION

For patients who have undergone treatment of primary melanoma, early detection of a local recurrence has important implications. An isolated local recurrence in a patient with favorable features can be treated with repeat wide local excision, with good oncologic outcomes. For these patients, long-term prognosis is not adversely affected by the local recurrence if it is detected and treated early, and 5-year survival continues to be a function of primary tumor thickness.[19,28,29] For those whose disease relapses in the regional lymph node basins, prognosis depends on the tumor burden at the time of detection, but early identification of regional recurrences and subsequent treatment with surgical resection can increase survival time compared with late identification of recurrences that present on clinical examination or with development of symptoms.[28] In the recently published final report from the landmark Multicenter Selective Lymphadenectomy Trial-1, Morton and colleagues[30] reported that for patients with intermediate-thickness melanoma, those who underwent nodal observation only and subsequently developed a clinically evident nodal recurrence had 5- and 10-year melanoma-specific survival rates of 57.5% and 41.5%, respectively, whereas patients with positive sentinel lymph node metastases found through biopsy and treated at original presentation had a 10-year melanoma-specific survival of 62.1%. The benefit of early detection of regional lymph node recurrences, therefore, highlights the importance of detecting them at a time when appropriate therapy still can be administered with curative intent.

For patients who develop distant melanoma recurrences, the appropriate therapeutic approach is highly debated. Because the lungs are the most common site of distant, metastatic melanoma involvement,[31] many patients undergo imaging studies aimed at detecting "treatable" distant recurrences. For patients with melanoma with pulmonary involvement, the 5-year overall survival is 4%.[32] For the 12% to 25% of patients who are candidates for surgical resection of their metastatic melanoma, 5-year survival may be modestly improved and is 30% in some studies.[32–34]

In a retrospective analysis of patients enrolled in the Multicenter Selective Lymphadenectomy Trial-1, Howard and colleagues[24] estimated that up to 50% of patients with stage IV melanoma may be candidates for surgical treatment of their metastatic disease. In that review, the median survival time was significantly longer for patients undergoing surgical resection of their metastatic disease (15.8 months) with or without systemic medical therapy than for patients who did not undergo surgery (6.9 months). The survival benefit was significantly greater among patients with a longer disease-free interval whose metastatic disease was isolated to one or two organ sites.[24] Therefore, although patient selection bias likely plays a large role in retrospective reports of survival after surgery for distant disease recurrence, a carefully selected subset of patients with advanced-stage melanoma would likely benefit from early detection of treatable metastatic disease and subsequent surgical intervention.

Because the early detection of melanoma recurrences has a potential survival benefit for a select population of patients, optimal surveillance strategies that can impact clinical care must be defined. The primary objective of surveillance should be to detect local, regional, and distant recurrences at a time when intervention can still improve survival. Note, however, that for the increasing numbers of melanoma survivors in the United States, no available data suggest that disease control, survival, or quality of life are significantly improved with routine surveillance imaging studies. Patients with local and regional recurrences, most of whom are diagnosed clinically, have favorable 5-year survival, as high as 80%.[22] Distant metastatic disease, however, which is usually diagnosed with routine oncologic surveillance imaging or imaging ordered as a result of symptom presentation, has uniformly poor 5-year survival once diagnosed (20% or less).[35] These data lead to the question of whether more intensive surveillance to detect recurrences before distant disease develops would translate to improved patient survival.

SURVEILLANCE EVALUATION MODALITIES

Clinical examination effectively diagnoses local recurrences in more than 50% of patients with treated melanoma in whom recurrent melanoma or second primary tumors develop.[28,36] In a study of 1062 patients with early stage melanoma (I-II), self-detection and clinical physical examination identified 95% of all recurrences at a median of 17 months following a sentinel lymph node biopsy with negative results.[37] A prospective database analysis of 118 patients with stage II or III melanoma found that 67% of recurrences were diagnosed through self-detection or symptomatic presentation. An additional 26% of recurrences were found by clinical examination on routine follow-up.[38] A review found that 18% of 38 patients with stage III melanoma developed a recurrence at a median disease-free interval of 25 months; most these recurrences (57%) were identified by the patient or physician in a clinical examination.[39]

Regional lymph node basins can be effectively evaluated using noninvasive ultrasonography. Studies have demonstrated that the sensitivity of ultrasonographic evaluation of the lymph node basins is 87% to 99%, with a specificity of 74% to 99%[39,40] when the tumors within the lymph node are greater than 1 mm.[41,42] To determine the effect of ultrasonographic surveillance in the detection of regional recurrences in patients with treated melanoma, a meta-analysis using data from a systematic review of four major medical indices was completed by Xing and colleagues.[43] For this analysis, patient-level data were extracted from the 74 studies deemed eligible using quality assessment and were subsequently modeled using Bayesian statistics to yield findings related to the sensitivity, specificity, and diagnostic odds ratio for imaging of the regional lymph nodes and of distant metastases using ultrasonography, CT, PET, and PET/CT, with confidence intervals (CIs) to define the posterior probability distribution for interval estimation. Ultrasonography had the highest sensitivity (60%; 95% CI, 33%–83%), specificity (97%; 95% CI, 88%–99%), and diagnostic odds ratio (42; 95% CI, 8.08–249.8) for the surveillance of regional lymph nodes.[43] Therefore, ultrasonography is superior to physical examination alone for the detection of regional lymph node recurrences[44,45]; as such, ultrasonography has been incorporated into many international guidelines for the follow-up of patients with melanoma.[46] The same study found that for the surveillance of distant metastases, PET/CT had the highest sensitivity (80%; 95% CI, 53%–9%3), specificity (87%; 95% CI, 54%–97%), and diagnostic odds ratio (1675; 95% CI, 226.5–15,920). Summary findings for this study appear in **Table 1**.

In the only prospective study evaluating surveillance for patients with melanoma according to stage, Garbe and colleagues[28] followed a cohort of 3008 patients with stage I-IV melanoma over a 2-year period. Patients were evaluated according to German surveillance guidelines, with frequent physical examinations (every 3 months) and routine ultrasonographic evaluation of the tumor scar and draining lymph node basins (annually for patients with stage I disease, every 6 months for those with stage II disease, and every 3–6 months for those with stage III disease). Cross-sectional imaging with CT scan or MRI was used only to evaluate suspicious clinical or ultrasonographic findings. Nearly 50% of recurrences were detected with clinical examination alone, even in patients with stage III disease. The addition of CT performed based on clinical suspicion detected an additional 27.7% of recurrences.[28]

SURVEILLANCE EFFECTIVENESS

To understand the extent to which surveillance imaging translates to a survival benefit for patients with treated melanoma, Rueth and colleagues[47] developed a decision-support model designed to evaluate the effectiveness of routine CT and PET/CT

Table 1
Surveillance strategies for patients with melanoma

Location and Imaging Method	% Median Sensitivity (95% Confidence Interval)	% Median Specificity (95% Confidence Interval)	Median Diagnostic Odds Ratio (95% Confidence Interval)
Regional lymph nodes			
Ultrasonography	96 (85–99)	99 (95–100)	1675 (226–15,920)
CT	61 (15–93)	97 (70–100)	46 (2–1354)
PET	87 (67–96)	98 (93–100)	391 (68–2737)
PET/CT	65 (20–93)	99 (92–100)	196 (11–4675)
Distant sites			
CT	63 (46–77)	78 (58–90)	6 (2–18)
PET	82 (72–88)	83 (70–91)	22 (9–51)
PET/CT	86 (76–93)	91 (79–97)	67 (20–230)

Adapted from Xing Y, Bronstein Y, Ross MI, et al. Contemporary diagnostic imaging modalities for the staging and surveillance of melanoma patients: a meta-analysis. J Natl Cancer Inst 2011;103:136; and Xing Y, Cromwell KD, Cormier JN. Review of diagnostic imaging modalities for the surveillance of melanoma patients. Dermatol Res Pract 2012;2012:3.

surveillance of patients with stage I-III melanoma. In this study, a probabilistic Markov model representing the stage-specific natural history of surgically treated melanoma was developed (**Fig. 2**). The model estimates were derived from 1600 patients with melanoma who were evaluated and surgically treated at a single institution. Patient-level time-to-event data were used to determine the monthly transition probabilities, which were estimated using parametric survival models from the time of definitive local/regional treatment. The study evaluated the ability of various surveillance imaging modalities and timelines (CT or PET/CT performed every 6 or 12 months for 5 years) to detect regional or distant recurrences that could be treated with surgical resection

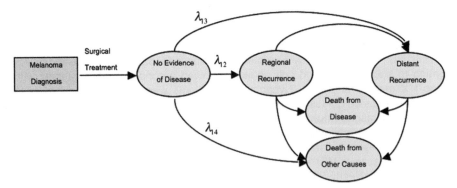

Fig. 2. Markov model representing the stage-specific natural history of surgically treated melanoma. Time horizon: lifetime. λ_{12} indicates monthly transition rate from no evidence of disease (NED) to regional recurrence; λ_{13}, monthly transition rate from NED to distant recurrence; λ_{14}, monthly transition rate from NED to death from other causes; $\lambda_1 = \lambda_{12} + \lambda_{13} + \lambda_{14}$ = monthly transition rate of NED. (*From* Rueth NM, Xing Y, Chiang YJ, et al. Is surveillance imaging effective for detecting surgically treatable recurrences in patients with melanoma? A comparative analysis of stage-specific surveillance strategies. Ann Surg 2014;259(6):1216, with permission.)

with curative intent, using established sensitivity and specificity data for contemporary diagnostic imaging modalities including CT, PET/CT, MRI, and ultrasound.[47]

For patients with stage I melanoma, in whom recurrence rates are low, the authors calculated that if routine surveillance imaging were performed at 12-month intervals, 362 CT scans or 249 PET/CT scans would have to be performed over the course of 5 years to diagnose one treatable recurrence in a patient with stage I disease.[47] Furthermore, they reported that routine annual surveillance imaging for patients with stage I melanoma would result in a 5-year total of 45,296 CT scans or 45,314 PET/CT scans per 10,000 patients to detect one treatable recurrence.

In contrast, as the incidence of regional or distant recurrence increased with disease stage, so too did the number of surgically treatable recurrences detected with routine surveillance imaging increase with stage. Among the highest-risk patients (those with stage IIIC disease) the authors calculated that routine surveillance CT or PET/CT performed every 12 months would detect surgically treatable regional and distant recurrence in 6.4% and 8.4% more patients, respectively, than would annual physical examination alone. In this population, 1 of every 34 CT scans and 1 of every 26 PET/CT scans would detect a treatable recurrence.

According to these identification estimations, although more treatable recurrences were detected with the use of routine PET/CT than with CT alone, there were no differences between CT and PET/CT in the calculated 5-year disease-specific survival, regardless of disease stage. Similarly, more frequent imaging (every 6 months vs every 12 months) did not substantially increase the 5-year disease-specific survival, regardless of disease stage (**Table 2**). The greatest survival benefit from more frequent

Table 2
Unadjusted 5-year disease-free survival, disease-specific survival, and increase in life expectancy with surveillance imaging

Stage/ Modality	6-mo Examination Interval			12-mo Examination Interval		
	5-y NED (%)	5-y DSS (%)	Average Increase in Life Expectancy (mo)	5-y NED (%)	5-y DSS (%)	Average Increase in Life Expectancy (mo)
Stage I						
CT	87.7	91.8	0.3	87.7	91.5	0.2
PET/CT	87.7	91.9	0.4	87.7	91.5	0.2
Stage II						
CT	70.5	77.0	0.9	70.5	76.2	0.5
PET/CT	70.5	77.4	1.1	70.5	76.3	0.5
Stage IIIA						
CT	72.0	76.1	0.8	72.0	75.7	0.4
PET/CT	72.0	76.3	0.9	72.0	75.8	0.4
Stage IIIB						
CT	48.3	52.9	1.4	48.3	52.4	0.7
PET/CT	48.3	53.4	1.7	48.3	52.5	0.7
Stage IIIC						
CT	32.1	37.0	1.8	32.1	36.4	0.8
PET/CT	32.1	37.6	2.0	32.1	36.5	0.8

Abbreviations: DSS, disease-specific survival; NED, no evidence of disease.
Adapted from Rueth NM, Xing Y, Chiang YJ, et al. Is surveillance imaging effective for detecting surgically treatable recurrences in patients with melanoma? A comparative analysis of stage-specific surveillance strategies. Ann Surg 2014;259(6):1219; with permission.

imaging was seen for patients with stage IIIB or IIIC disease. Even in these groups, however, the difference between a less rigorous imaging strategy of CT every 12 months and a more rigorous imaging strategy of PET/CT every 6 months in terms of 5-year disease-specific survival was minimal.

Notably, routine surveillance imaging did not substantially increase life expectancy for any subgroup of patients with melanoma regardless of imaging modality or frequency (**Fig. 3**). For patients with stage I melanoma, in whom the average life expectancy was 51.6 months without surveillance imaging, the increase in life expectancy that resulted from the addition of rigorous, routine surveillance PET/CT imaging every 6 months was only 0.4 months. This translated to an increase in relative survival time (relative to the survival of patients who underwent clinical examination alone) of only 0.7%. Even for patients with stage IIIC disease who underwent the most aggressive imaging strategy of PET/CT surveillance imaging every 6 months and in whom treatable recurrence rates exceeded 20%, the mean increase in life expectancy was only 2 months (from 30.0 to 32.0 months), which translated to a relative survival time increase of 6.8%.

With a negative predictive value nearing 100%, routine imaging can effectively rule out melanoma recurrence; however, the high rate of false-positive studies and the low positive predictive value associated with imaging mean that many studies must be performed to detect a small number of treatable recurrences, likely with little impact on patient survival.[48] Even the identification of treatable recurrent disease by means of routine surveillance imaging using the most sensitive tests available would likely result in only a minimal increase in life expectancy compared with results for routine clinical examination alone. For patients with stage III melanoma, the average gain in absolute life expectancy as a result of routine surveillance imaging is only a few months. These data solidify the point that for most patients with surgically treated melanoma, routine imaging is not likely to offer a substantial long-term survival benefit; however, a subset of stage III patients may obtain a modest survival benefit from routine surveillance imaging.

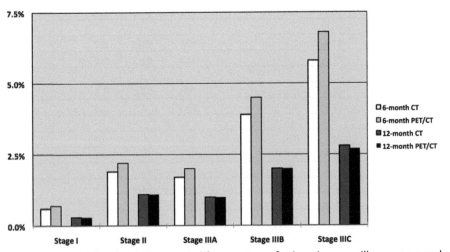

Fig. 3. Stage-specific relative increase in life expectancy for imaging surveillance compared with clinical examination alone (by stage and frequency). (*From* Rueth NM, Xing Y, Chiang YJ, et al. Is surveillance imaging effective for detecting surgically treatable recurrences in patients with melanoma? A comparative analysis of stage-specific surveillance strategies. Ann Surg 2014;259(6):1220, with permission.)

VARIATION IN CURRENT SURVEILLANCE PRACTICES

In the absence of evidence-based guidelines, many clinicians use practice patterns that they or their patients are most comfortable with. To identify the most commonly used frequency, duration, and type of follow-up for patients with melanoma, Cromwell and colleagues[49] completed a systematic review of three medical indices and found significant variability in surveillance practices depending on the country where the study was conducted and the background of the treating clinician. A total of 104 studies were eligible for inclusion in that review, encompassing studies done in seven countries (Australia/New Zealand, Canada, Germany, United Kingdom, United States, the Netherlands, and Switzerland [**Table 3**]) and studies with treating clinicians in four medical specialties (general practitioner, dermatologist, medical oncologist, and surgical oncologist [**Table 4**]). Practices varied between country of location and type of specialist.

In the review of Cromwell and colleagues,[49] among patients with stage I melanoma, intervals between visits during the first 2 years after treatment ranged from every 2 months to every 12 months, with routine imaging that often included lymph node ultrasonography and chest x-ray radiography. Thereafter, in the absence of recurrence, visit intervals decreased to 3 to 12 months for years 3 to 5 after treatment. The highest frequencies of visits were seen in the United Kingdom and the Netherlands.[49] General practitioners evaluated patients more frequently than clinicians in any other specialty.

As reported in Cromwell and colleagues,[49] for patients with stage II melanoma, clinical examination frequency was less varied, with clinicians in most countries screening these patients at least every 3 months. Clinicians in Canada, the United States, and Switzerland reported common use of CT scans of the chest, abdomen, and pelvis area, and clinicians in Germany frequently used MRI in addition to CT. All specialists routinely evaluated patients every 3 months for the first 3 years after diagnosis. After 3 years of disease-free survival, surgical oncologists tended to decrease patients' clinical visits to every 6 months, whereas other specialists continued with visits at 3-month intervals through year 5.[49]

For patients with stage III melanoma, in whom the risk of recurrence is considerably higher than in those with earlier-stage disease, variation in type and frequency of follow-up remains high. Among most specialties and countries, the use of diagnostic imaging tools was much more widespread, with ultrasonography being the most commonly used strategy, followed by PET/CT and CT alone (see **Tables 3** and **4**; **Table 5**).[49]

COSTS OF SURVEILLANCE

Such extreme variations in clinical practice and resource use when these variations likely have a minimal impact on life expectancy have important implications for clinical care, particularly in the contemporary era of increasing cost-consciousness in health care. Hofmann and colleagues[50] reported that in Germany, imaging studies detected 25% of melanoma recurrences but accounted for 50% of follow-up costs. The cost per detected first recurrence in patients with stage I disease was as high as €35,900 ($32,310 according to 2002 conversion data) for aggressive imaging regimens, whereas the cost per detected, treatable metastases using clinical examination alone ranged from €2800 ($2520) for patients with stage III disease to €13,300 ($11,970) in patients with stage I-II recurrence in 2002.[50] Importantly, in this study, there was no survival difference between patients with recurrences detected by clinical examination and patients with asymptomatic recurrences detected with imaging.[48] Similarly, Basseres and colleagues[51] concluded that for patients with

Table 3
Stage-specific surveillance guidelines by country during years 1 to 5

Stage/Means of Detection	Australia/New Zealand[63-65]	Canada[66]	Germany[67-70]	United Kingdom[71-73]	United States[1,36,74-76]	The Netherlands[77-80]	Switzerland[81,82]
Number of visits per year							
Stage I							
Years 1–2	1–2	2–4	3–4	2–6	1–3	3–4	2
Year 3	1–2	2–4	3–4	2–3	1–3	3–4	2
Years 4–5	1–2	2–4	2	1–2	1–3	4–5	1–2
Stage II							
Years 1–2	1–4	4	2–4	4	2–4	3	2–4
Year 3	1–4	4	2–4	2	1–4	3	2–4
Years 4–5	1–4	2	2–4	2	1–4	2	2–3
Stage III							
Years 1–2	2–4	4	2–4	4	2–4	4	4
Year 3	2–4	4	2–4	2	1–4	4	4
Years 4–5	2–4	2	2–4	2	1–4	4	2
Recommended evaluations							
Self-examination	Yes	Yes	Yes	Yes	Yes	Yes	Yes
Routine diagnostic imaging							

Stage I	No	Sonography of regional nodal basin	No	Photography, abdominal sonography, chest radiography	Chest radiograph	No	Chest radiograph, sonography of regional nodal basin
Stage II	Sonography of regional nodal basin	Chest radiograph, bone and liver-spleen scan	Chest radiograph, CT/MRI, and PET	Photography, abdominal sonography, chest radiography	Chest radiograph, CT of chest, abdomen and pelvis	No	Sonography of regional nodal basin, PET or CT
Stage III	Sonography of regional nodal basin	Chest radiograph, bone and liver-spleen scan	Chest radiograph, CT/MRI, PET	Clinical photography, abdominal sonography, chest radiography	PET/CT	No	Sonography of regional nodal basin, PET or CT
Symptom-initiated					Chest radiography, PET, CT, MRI, PET/CT		Abdominal sonography, CT, MRI, PET/CT (for non-stage III)
Laboratory assessment	No	CBC, liver function test	S100 serum protein (≥stage 2)	CBC, liver function, creatinine, lactate dehydrogenase	No	No	S-100 serum protein (≥stage II)

Abbreviation: CBC, complete blood count.

Adapted from Cromwell KD, Ross MI, Xing Y, et al. Variability in melanoma post-treatment surveillance practices by country and physician specialty: a systematic review. Melanoma Res 2012;22:380; with permission.

Table 4
Stage-specific surveillance guidelines by physician specialty during years 1–5

Stage/Means of Detection	General Practitioner[83–89]	Dermatologist[68,90,91]	Medical Oncologist[70,90]	Surgical Oncologist[38,79]
Number of visits per year				
Stage I	4	2	2	NA
Stage II				
Years 1–2	4	4	4	4
Year 3	4	4	4	4
Years 4–5	4	4	4	2
Stage III	4	4	4	4 (years 1–3) 2 (years 4–5)
Recommended evaluations				
Self-examination	Yes	Yes	Yes	Yes
Routine diagnostic imaging	No	CT for stage III	Sonography of regional lymph nodes	CT of chest, abdomen, and pelvis
Laboratory assessment	No	LDH, AP, protein S-100β	LDH, AP	CBC, LDH (>stage II)

Abbreviations: AP, alkaline phosphatase; CBC, complete blood count; LDH, lactate dehydrogenase; NA, not available.

Adapted from Cromwell KD, Ross MI, Xing Y, et al. Variability in melanoma post-treatment surveillance practices by country and physician specialty: a systematic review. Melanoma Res 2012;22:389; with permission.

Table 5
Stage-specific recommendations for number of surveillance visits per year after year 5

Country/Specialty	Stage		
	I	II	III
By country			
Australia/New Zealand[63–65]	1	1	1
Canada[66]	1	1	1
Germany[67–70,92]	1–2	1–2	2
United Kingdom[71–73]	As needed	As needed	As needed
United States[1,74]	1	1	1
Switzerland[81]	1	1	1
The Netherlands[77–80]	1	1	1
By physician specialty			
Dermatologist[68,90,91]	1	1–2	2
General practitioner[83–89]	1	1	1
Medical oncologist[70,90]	1–2	1–2	2
Surgical oncologist[38,79]	1	1	1

Adapted from Cromwell KD, Ross MI, Xing Y, et al. Variability in melanoma post-treatment surveillance practices by country and physician specialty: a systematic review. Melanoma Res 2012;22:381; with permission.

stage I melanoma treated in France, clinical examination was the only cost-effective surveillance modality. Hengge and colleagues[52] calculated that for patients with stage II disease, the median cost to detect a recurrence with clinical examination was €2715 ($2444); this cost increased to €32,007 ($28,806) when surveillance imaging was added. All of these investigators concluded that routine surveillance imaging for patients with surgically treated stage I or II melanoma is not cost-effective.

To understand the potential role of imaging for patients with more advanced disease, Bastiaannet and colleagues[53] conducted a multi-institutional, multinational cost analysis exploring the utility of cross-sectional imaging for preoperative staging for patients presenting with clinically detectable nodal disease. In their study, the addition of CT decreased the cost of staging and subsequent treatment by 5.5% compared with chest radiography and clinical examination alone, whereas the addition of PET/CT to chest radiography and clinical examination increased these costs by 15.1%.[51] This cost difference was because PET/CT, which has a slightly higher diagnostic accuracy than CT, upstaged disease, which led to higher adjuvant treatment costs despite lower surgical treatment costs. The authors concluded that routine preoperative imaging in patients with melanoma presenting with clinically detectable regional metastases (stage III) is cost-effective. However, they could not make inferences about postoperative surveillance imaging because of the study design.[51] In fact, the cost-effectiveness and clinical impact of routine postoperative surveillance imaging for patients with stage III disease has not been well evaluated in any contemporary studies; an analysis that critically explores the diagnostic and survival benefits of postoperative surveillance imaging in these patients in the context of resource use and medical costs is needed.

Clearly, investigations designed to develop standardized follow-up protocols for melanoma cancer survivors that balance cost, resource use, and patient outcomes are very much needed; such studies are currently ongoing.

OTHER PRACTICE IMPLICATIONS

Although the early detection of a surgically resectable recurrence may be the primary reason for performing routine surveillance imaging, other ramifications of surveillance must be considered. Surveillance also can lead to reassurance or confirmation of an ongoing disease-free interval, which could not only guide future surveillance but also benefit quality of life, the initiation of systemic treatment of nonsurgical candidates or early enrollment into clinical trials, and the detection of new primary malignancies or second primary melanomas.[47,49,50]

In a recent meta-analysis of 15 survey-based studies evaluating the psychosocial response to melanoma, Rychetnik and colleagues[54] reported that despite increasing evidence refuting the benefits of routine surveillance imaging for patients with early stage disease, clinicians continue to order surveillance imaging studies for patients with stage I and II disease to provide reassurance. Nearly 75% of such patients in that study underwent a wide range of diagnostic imaging studies (conventional chest radiography, CT, or ultrasonography) that are not currently recommended by published guidelines; the authors noted that one of the primary reasons that physicians ordered diagnostic tests was patient anxiety or patient request.[52] This aggressive use of surveillance imaging suggests a need for ongoing, data-driven initiatives that aim to mitigate anxiety and improve survivor quality of life by delineating when surveillance imaging can provide actual survival benefit while reducing potentially unnecessary cost.

Less aggressive surveillance also may reduce adverse effects caused by imaging procedures. Imaging studies are not without risk to the patient, with the potential for contrast dye reactions, renal injury, and harmful radiation exposure. Radiation exposure is a potential consideration for clinicians ordering surveillance imaging studies for melanoma survivors. Mathews and colleagues[55] recently estimated that radiation exposure is associated with an excess incidence rate of 9.38 cancers per 100,000 person-years at risk. Similarly, Miglioretti and colleagues[56] studied radiation exposure resulting from CT imaging in children and projected that the 4 million pediatric CT scans performed annually in the United States would result in 4870 future malignancies. Although the risks of radiation exposure are less well studied in adults, the American College of Radiology has developed a series of guidelines to help identify the clinical conditions in which imaging is most appropriate,[57] and the National Institute of Biomedical Imaging and Bioengineering is challenging investigators to develop new technology that will drastically reduce radiation exposure resulting from radiographic imaging.[58]

Once patients are diagnosed with disease recurrence, the limited ability of systemic therapy to offer a long-term survival benefit for patients has been a vexing challenge for melanoma care providers, resulting in a heavy reliance on surgical treatment. Recent studies have shown promising results using targeted systemic therapies and combination therapies in the treatment of unresectable stage III and stage IV disease.[59,60] The promising early results seen for patients treated with novel targeted agents, such as vemurafinib and ipilimumab, has resulted in rapid changes in the landscape of systemic melanoma treatment. It is possible, therefore, that future therapeutic developments will result in increasingly effective systemic treatment options for patients with recurrent disease and that a subset of these patients will derive a survival benefit from early detection of disease recurrence. In the meantime, as rapid advances are being made in the areas of targeted therapies, vaccine trials, and innovative treatments combining traditional interleukin or cytotoxic chemotherapy agents with novel drugs, the identification of patients with locoregional melanoma recurrence who are appropriate candidates for enrollment into clinical trials must be considered when choosing individualized patient surveillance strategies.

In addition to the risk of locoregional or distant melanoma recurrence, we must not overlook the risk of patients with treated melanoma developing a second primary melanoma or other primary malignancy. Recent conditional survival analyses have demonstrated that the ongoing risk of dying of a treated melanoma decreases as survival time increases[48,61]; however, the risk of developing a second primary malignancy increases over time. This risk is substantial; in a retrospective review using the Surveillance, Epidemiology, and End Results database, Spanogle and colleagues[62] found that among 16,591 patients with previously treated melanoma, the risk of developing a second primary malignancy was 32% higher than in the general population without a melanoma diagnosis. The risk was highest among patients younger than age 40 years, highlighting the need for ongoing dermatologic surveillance aimed at detecting second melanomas and for routine medical care and guideline-recommended cancer screening, including mammography and colonoscopy.

SUMMARY

Cumulative findings support the current National Comprehensive Cancer Network guidelines for surveillance in early stage melanoma (stages IA-IIA), which recommend lifelong dermatologic surveillance with regular comprehensive skin examinations, adding imaging studies only if there is clinical suspicion of recurrence.[1] Regular clinical examination offers the highest diagnostic yield in detecting melanoma recurrences, with additional diagnostic benefit seen when imaging is used for patients in whom clinical evaluation or symptomatic presentation suggests the presence of distant disease.

However, for patients with locally or regionally advanced melanoma (stages IIB-IIIC), there is a paucity of data to support the use of rigorous, routine surveillance imaging studies following appropriate staging and surgical treatment of their disease. Contemporary guidelines recommend, based on low-level evidence (category 2B), that clinicians consider the addition of CT and/or PET/CT every 3 to 12 months for these patients.[1] However, current data indicate that such a regimen would result in an exceedingly large number of studies performed to detect a limited number of surgically treatable recurrences and would have little impact on patient survival. Although there likely is a subset of patients with high-risk melanoma in whom routine oncologic imaging surveillance has the potential to offer survival benefit, a more judicious approach to the use of imaging studies may be equally effective with little detrimental impact on survival. Such considerations are of increasing interest in the modern era of rising health care costs and impending limitations on resource use.

REFERENCES

1. NCCN Clinical Practice Guidelines in Oncology: Melanoma, 2010. Available at: http://www.nccn.org/professionals/physician_gls/f_guidelines.asp.
2. Ohlsson B, Breland U, Ekberg H, et al. Follow-up after curative surgery for colorectal carcinoma. Randomized comparison with no follow-up. Dis Colon Rectum 1995;38:619–26.
3. Pietra N, Sarli L, Costi R, et al. Role of follow-up in management of local recurrences of colorectal cancer: a prospective, randomized study. Dis Colon Rectum 1998;41:1127–33.
4. Rodriguez-Moranta F, Salo J, Arcusa A, et al. Postoperative surveillance in patients with colorectal cancer who have undergone curative resection: a prospective, multicenter, randomized, controlled trial. J Clin Oncol 2006;24: 386–93.
5. Schoemaker D, Black R, Giles L, et al. Yearly colonoscopy, liver CT, and chest radiography do not influence 5-year survival of colorectal cancer patients. Gastroenterology 1998;114:7–14.
6. Secco GB, Fardelli R, Gianquinto D, et al. Efficacy and cost of risk-adapted follow-up in patients after colorectal cancer surgery: a prospective, randomized and controlled trial. Eur J Surg Oncol 2002;28:418–23.
7. Kjeldsen BJ, Kronborg O, Fenger C, et al. A prospective randomized study of follow-up after radical surgery for colorectal cancer. Br J Surg 1997;84:666–9.
8. Makela JT, Laitinen SO, Kairaluoma MI. Five-year follow-up after radical surgery for colorectal cancer. Results of a prospective randomized trial. Arch Surg 1995; 130:1062–7.
9. Renehan AG, Egger M, Saunders MP, et al. Impact on survival of intensive follow up after curative resection for colorectal cancer: systematic review and meta-analysis of randomised trials. BMJ 2002;324:813.
10. Rosen M, Chan L, Beart RW Jr, et al. Follow-up of colorectal cancer: a meta-analysis. Dis Colon Rectum 1998;41:1116–26.
11. Impact of follow-up testing on survival and health-related quality of life in breast cancer patients. A multicenter randomized controlled trial. The GIVIO investigators. JAMA 1994;271:1587–92.
12. Margenthaler JA, Johnson FE, Cyr AE. Intensity of follow-up after breast cancer surgery: low versus high? Ann Surg Oncol 2014;21:733–7.

13. Michela WA. Physician remuneration has impact on hospital costs. Hospitals 1977;51:30–4.
14. Rosselli Del Turco M, Palli D, Cariddi A, et al. Intensive diagnostic follow-up after treatment of primary breast cancer. A randomized trial. National Research Council Project on Breast Cancer follow-up. JAMA 1994;271:1593–7.
15. Siegel R, Ward E, Brawley O, et al. Cancer statistics, 2011: the impact of eliminating socioeconomic and racial disparities on premature cancer deaths. CA Cancer J Clin 2011;61:212–36.
16. Siegel R, Ma J, Zou Z, et al. Cancer statistics, 2014. CA Cancer J Clin 2014;64: 9–29.
17. Leiter U, Meier F, Schittek B, et al. The natural course of cutaneous melanoma. J Surg Oncol 2004;86:172–8.
18. MacCormack MA, Cohen LM, Rogers GS. Local melanoma recurrence: a clarification of terminology. Dermatol Surg 2004;30:1533–8.
19. Benvenuto-Andrade C, Oseitutu A, Agero AL, et al. Cutaneous melanoma: surveillance of patients for recurrence and new primary melanomas. Dermatol Ther 2005;18:423–35.
20. Soong SJ, Harrison RA, McCarthy WH, et al. Factors affecting survival following local, regional, or distant recurrence from localized melanoma. J Surg Oncol 1998;67:228–33.
21. Dicker TJ, Kavanagh GM, Herd RM, et al. A rational approach to melanoma follow-up in patients with primary cutaneous melanoma. Br J Dermatol 1999; 140:249–54.
22. Crowley NJ, Seigler HF. Late recurrence of malignant melanoma. Analysis of 168 patients. Ann Surg 1990;212:173–7.
23. Petersen RP, Hanish SI, Haney JC, et al. Improved survival with pulmonary metastasectomy: an analysis of 1720 patients with pulmonary metastatic melanoma. J Thorac Cardiovasc Surg 2007;133:104–10.
24. Howard JH, Thompson JF, Mozzillo N, et al. Metastasectomy for distant metastatic melanoma: analysis of data from the first Multicenter Selective Lymphadenectomy Trial (MSLT-I). Ann Surg Oncol 2012;19:2547–55.
25. Young SE, Martinez SR, Essner R. The role of surgery in treatment of stage IV melanoma. J Surg Oncol 2006;94:344–51.
26. Riker AI, Kirksey L, Thompson L, et al. Current surgical management of melanoma. Expert Rev Anticancer Ther 2006;6:1569–83.
27. Romano E, Scordo M, Dusza SW, et al. Site and timing of first relapse in stage III melanoma patients: implications for follow-up guidelines. J Clin Oncol 2010;28: 3042–7.
28. Garbe C, Paul A, Kohler-Spath H, et al. Prospective evaluation of a follow-up schedule in cutaneous melanoma patients: recommendations for an effective follow-up strategy. J Clin Oncol 2003;21:520–9.
29. Rhodes AR. Cutaneous melanoma and intervention strategies to reduce tumor-related mortality: what we know, what we don't know, and what we think we know that isn't so. Dermatol Ther 2006;19:50–69.
30. Morton DL, Thompson JF, Cochran AJ, et al. Final trial report of sentinel-node biopsy versus nodal observation in melanoma. N Engl J Med 2014;370:599–609.
31. Wong CY, Helm MA, Helm TN, et al. Patterns of skin metastases: a review of 25 years' experience at a single cancer center. Int J Dermatol 2014;53:56–60.
32. Harpole DH Jr, Johnson CM, Wolfe WG, et al. Analysis of 945 cases of pulmonary metastatic melanoma. J Thorac Cardiovasc Surg 1992;103:743–8 [discussion: 748–50].

33. Coit DG. Role of surgery for metastatic malignant melanoma: a review. Semin Surg Oncol 1993;9:239–45.

34. Wong JH, Euhus DM, Morton DL. Surgical resection for metastatic melanoma to the lung. Arch Surg 1988;123:1091–5.

35. Tsao H, Cosimi AB, Sober AJ. Ultra-late recurrence (15 years or longer) of cutaneous melanoma. Cancer 1997;79:2361–70.

36. Romero JB, Stefanato CM, Kopf AW, et al. Follow-up recommendations for patients with stage I malignant melanoma. J Dermatol Surg Oncol 1994;20:175–8.

37. Moore Dalal K, Zhou Q, Panageas KS, et al. Methods of detection of first recurrence in patients with stage I/II primary cutaneous melanoma after sentinel lymph node biopsy. Ann Surg Oncol 2008;15:2206–14.

38. Meyers MO, Yeh JJ, Frank J, et al. Method of detection of initial recurrence of stage II/III cutaneous melanoma: analysis of the utility of follow-up staging. Ann Surg Oncol 2009;16:941–7.

39. Baker JJ, Meyers MO, Frank J, et al. Routine restaging PET/CT and detection of initial recurrence in sentinel lymph node positive stage III melanoma. Am J Surg 2014;207:549–54.

40. Tregnaghi A, De Candia A, Calderone M, et al. Ultrasonographic evaluation of superficial lymph node metastases in melanoma. Eur J Radiol 1997;24:216–21.

41. Solivetti FM, Elia F, Santaguida MG, et al. The role of ultrasound and ultrasound-guided fine needle aspiration biopsy of lymph nodes in patients with skin tumours. Radiol Oncol 2014;48:29–34.

42. Voit CA, van Akkooi AC, Schafer-Hesterberg G, et al. Rotterdam Criteria for sentinel node (SN) tumor burden and the accuracy of ultrasound (US)-guided fine-needle aspiration cytology (FNAC): can US-guided FNAC replace SN staging in patients with melanoma? J Clin Oncol 2009;27:4994–5000.

43. Xing Y, Bronstein Y, Ross MI, et al. Contemporary diagnostic imaging modalities for the staging and surveillance of melanoma patients: a meta-analysis. J Natl Cancer Inst 2011;103:129–42.

44. Bafounta ML, Beauchet A, Chagnon S, et al. Ultrasonography or palpation for detection of melanoma nodal invasion: a meta-analysis. Lancet Oncol 2004;5:673–80.

45. Voit C, Mayer T, Kron M, et al. Efficacy of ultrasound B-scan compared with physical examination in follow-up of melanoma patients. Cancer 2001;91:2409–16.

46. Ulrich J, van Akkooi AJ, Eggermont AM, et al. New developments in melanoma: utility of ultrasound imaging (initial staging, follow-up and pre-SLNB). Expert Rev Anticancer Ther 2011;11:1693–701.

47. Rueth NM, Xing Y, Chiang YJ, et al. Is surveillance imaging effective for detecting surgically treatable recurrences in patients with melanoma? A comparative analysis of stage-specific surveillance strategies. Ann Surg 2014;259(6):1215–22.

48. Rueth NM, Groth SS, Tuttle TM, et al. Conditional survival after surgical treatment of melanoma: an analysis of the Surveillance, Epidemiology, and End Results database. Ann Surg Oncol 2010;17:1662–8.

49. Cromwell KD, Ross MI, Xing Y, et al. Variability in melanoma post-treatment surveillance practices by country and physician specialty: a systematic review. Melanoma Res 2012;22:376–85.

50. Hofmann U, Szedlak M, Rittgen W, et al. Primary staging and follow-up in melanoma patients: monocenter evaluation of methods, costs and patient survival. Br J Cancer 2002;87:151–7.

51. Basseres N, Grob JJ, Richard MA, et al. Cost-effectiveness of surveillance of stage I melanoma. A retrospective appraisal based on a 10-year experience in a dermatology department in France. Dermatology 1995;191:199–203.

52. Hengge UR, Wallerand A, Stutzki A, et al. Cost-effectiveness of reduced follow-up in malignant melanoma. J Dtsch Dermatol Ges 2007;5:898–907.
53. Bastiaannet E, Uyl-de Groot CA, Brouwers AH, et al. Cost-effectiveness of adding FDG-PET or CT to the diagnostic work-up of patients with stage III melanoma. Ann Surg 2012;255:771–6.
54. Rychetnik L, McCaffery K, Morton R, et al. Psychosocial aspects of post-treatment follow-up for stage I/II melanoma: a systematic review of the literature. Psychooncology 2013;22(4):721–36.
55. Mathews JD, Forsythe AV, Brady Z, et al. Cancer risk in 680 000 people exposed to computed tomography scans in childhood or adolescence: data linkage study of 11 million Australians. BMJ 2013;346:f2360.
56. Miglioretti DL, Johnson E, Williams A, et al. The use of computed tomography in pediatrics and the associated radiation exposure and estimated cancer risk. JAMA Pediatr 2013;167(8):700–7.
57. Stern EJ, Adam EJ, Bettman MA, et al. Proceedings from the first global summit on radiological quality and safety. J Am Coll Radiol 2014;11(10):959–67.
58. Goodman DM. Initiatives focus on limiting radiation exposure to patients during CT scans. JAMA 2013;309:647–8.
59. Chapman PB, Hauschild A, Robert C, et al. Improved survival with vemurafenib in melanoma with BRAF V600E mutation. N Engl J Med 2011;364:2507–16.
60. Hodi FS, O'Day SJ, McDermott DF, et al. Improved survival with ipilimumab in patients with metastatic melanoma. N Engl J Med 2010;363:711–23.
61. Xing Y, Chang GJ, Hu CY, et al. Conditional survival estimates improve over time for patients with advanced melanoma: results from a population-based analysis. Cancer 2010;116:2234–41.
62. Spanogle JP, Clarke CA, Aroner S, et al. Risk of second primary malignancies following cutaneous melanoma diagnosis: a population-based study. J Am Acad Dermatol 2010;62:757–67.
63. Australian-Cancer-Network-Melanoma-Guidelines-Revision-Working-Party. Clinical practice guidelines for the management of melanoma in Australia and New Zealand. In: Network CCAaAC, editor. Wellington (New Zealand): Sydney and New Zealand Guidelines Group; 2008.
64. Thompson JF, Shaw HM, Stretch JR, et al. The Sydney melanoma unit: a multidisciplinary melanoma treatment center. Surg Clin North Am 2003;83:431–51.
65. Francken AB, Accortt NA, Shaw HM, et al. Follow-up schedules after treatment for malignant melanoma. Br J Surg 2008;95:1401–7.
66. Kersey PA, Iscoe NA, Gapski JA, et al. The value of staging and serial follow-up investigations in patients with completely resected, primary, cutaneous malignant melanoma. Br J Surg 1985;72:614–7.
67. Garbe C, Hauschild A, Volkenandt M, et al. Evidence and interdisciplinary consensus-based German guidelines: diagnosis and surveillance of melanoma. Melanoma Res 2007;17:393–9.
68. Ugurel S, Enk A. Skin cancer: follow-up, rehabilitation, palliative and supportive care. J Dtsch Dermatol Ges 2008;6:492–8 [quiz: 499].
69. Dummer R, Hauschild A, Pentheroudakis G. Cutaneous malignant melanoma: ESMO clinical recommendations for diagnosis, treatment and follow-up. Ann Oncol 2009;20(Suppl 4):129–31.
70. Garbe C, Schadendorf D. Surveillance and follow-up examinations in cutaneous melanoma. Onkologie 2003;26:241–6.
71. Roberts DL, Anstey AV, Barlow RJ, et al. U.K. guidelines for the management of cutaneous melanoma. Br J Dermatol 2002;146:7–17.

72. Meier F, Will S, Ellwanger U, et al. Metastatic pathways and time courses in the orderly progression of cutaneous melanoma. Br J Dermatol 2002;147:62–70.
73. Marsden JR, Newton-Bishop JA, Burrows L, et al. Revised UK guidelines for the management of cutaneous melanoma 2010. J Plast Reconstr Aesthet Surg 2010; 63:1401–19.
74. Sober AJ, Chuang TY, Duvic M, et al. Guidelines of care for primary cutaneous melanoma. J Am Acad Dermatol 2001;45:579–86.
75. Chu D, Coit DG, Daud A, et al. Melanoma: treatment guidelines for patients (part 2). Dermatol Nurs 2005;17:191–8.
76. Olson JA Jr, Jaques DP, Coit DG, et al. Staging work-up and post-treatment surveillance of patients with melanoma. Clin Plast Surg 2000;27:377–90, viii.
77. Rumke P, van Everdingen JE. Consensus on the management of melanoma of the skin in The Netherlands. Dutch melanoma working party. Eur J Cancer 1992;28: 600–4.
78. Nieweg OE, Kroon BB. The conundrum of follow-up: should it be abandoned? Surg Oncol Clin N Am 2006;15:319–30.
79. Kroon BB, Nieweg OE, Hoekstra HJ, et al. Principles and guidelines for surgeons: management of cutaneous malignant melanoma. European Society of Surgical Oncology Brussels. Eur J Surg Oncol 1997;23:550–8.
80. Francken AB, Bastiaannet E, Hoekstra HJ. Follow-up in patients with localised primary cutaneous melanoma. Lancet Oncol 2005;6:608–21.
81. Dummer R, Panizzon R, Bloch PH, et al. Updated Swiss guidelines for the treatment and follow-up of cutaneous melanoma. Dermatology 2005;210:39–44.
82. Dummer R, Guggenheim M, Arnold AW, et al. Updated Swiss guidelines for the treatment and follow-up of cutaneous melanoma. Swiss Med Wkly 2011;141: w13320.
83. Murchie P, Hannaford PC, Wyke S, et al. Designing an integrated follow-up programme for people treated for cutaneous malignant melanoma: a practical application of the MRC framework for the design and evaluation of complex interventions to improve health. Fam Pract 2007;24:283–92.
84. Florey CV, Yule B, Fogg A, et al. A randomized trial of immediate discharge of surgical patients to general practice. J Public Health Med 1994;16:455–64.
85. Francken AB, Hoekstra-Weebers JW, Hoekstra HJ. Is GP-led follow-up feasible? Br J Cancer 2010;102:1445–6.
86. Murchie P. Environmental impact of GP-led melanoma follow up. Br J Gen Pract 2007;57:837–8.
87. Murchie P, Delaney EK, Campbell NC, et al. GP-led melanoma follow-up: the practical experience of GPs. Fam Pract 2009;26:317–24.
88. Murchie P, Delaney EK, Campbell NC, et al. GP-led melanoma follow-up: views and feelings of patient recipients. Support Care Cancer 2009;18:225–33.
89. Murchie P, Nicolson MC, Hannaford PC, et al. Patient satisfaction with GP-led melanoma follow-up: a randomised controlled trial. Br J Cancer 2010;102: 1447–55.
90. Brown MD. Office management of melanoma patients. Semin Cutan Med Surg 2010;29:232–7.
91. McGuire ST, Secrest AM, Andrulonis R, et al. Surveillance of patients for early detection of melanoma: patterns in dermatologist vs patient discovery. Arch Dermatol 2011;147:673–8.
92. Garbe C. A rational approach to the follow-up of melanoma patients. Recent Results Cancer Res 2002;160:205–15.

372.
373.
374.
375.
376.
377.

Moving?

Make sure your subscription moves with you!

To notify us of your new address, find your **Clinics Account Number** (located on your mailing label above your name), and contact customer service at:

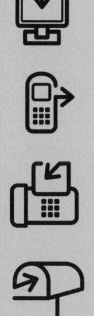

Email: journalscustomerservice-usa@elsevier.com

800-654-2452 (subscribers in the U.S. & Canada)
314-447-8871 (subscribers outside of the U.S. & Canada)

Fax number: 314-447-8029

Elsevier Health Sciences Division
Subscription Customer Service
3251 Riverport Lane
Maryland Heights, MO 63043

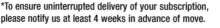

Printed and bound by CPI Group (UK) Ltd, Croydon, CR0 4YY

03/10/2024

01040491-0017